LABORATORY TESTS
in common use

laboratory tests
IN COMMON USE

by
SOLOMON GARB, M.D., F.A.C.P.
*Scientific Director, American Medical
Center at Denver*

FIFTH EDITION

 SPRINGER Publishing Company, Inc.
New York, N.Y.

Copyright © 1971

SPRINGER PUBLISHING COMPANY, INC.

200 Park Avenue South New York, N.Y. 10003

Fifth Edition, September 1971
Fourth Edition, November 1966
Third Edition, September 1963
Second Edition, September 1959
First Edition, April 1956

Library of Congress Catalog Card Number: 73-161127
Standard Book Number: 0-8261-0185-2, soft
0-8261-0186-0, hard

Current printing (last digit):
10 9 8 7 6 5 4 3 2

Printed in U.S.A.

Preface to Fifth Edition

This edition continues and expands the listings of drugs and foods that may interfere with laboratory tests to give misleading results. Unfortunately, our knowledge of such interferences is still limited, and there are probably many more situations in which drugs and foods can result in spurious laboratory test results.

Following suggestions from a number of readers, a separate section has been added to each laboratory test description, indicating food or drink restrictions. In earlier editions, this material had been included in the general discussion, but readers indicated that a separate section for ready reference would be helpful. Other suggestions from readers have been most helpful in improving this edition.

A few obsolete tests have been deleted, and twenty-four new tests have been added to bring the edition up to date.

I want to express my appreciation to Vincent Lagerborg, M.D., Ph.D., Chief of Pathology at American Medical Center at Denver for his review of the manuscript and many helpful suggestions. I am also grateful to Mrs. Martha Morris for her efficient secretarial help.

August 1971   SOLOMON GARB, M.D.

Contents

1

Introduction

Laboratory tests aid in the diagnosis and management of various disorders. Only those in relatively common use are included in this book. A test may be ordered by a physician to confirm his suspicion or impression, or it may be performed routinely on most or all patients. Routine tests are carried out because the disorders they demonstrate are relatively common and the tests themselves relatively easy to perform. An example of this sort of test is the determination of blood hemoglobin concentration. A substantial proportion of the population has anemia, so that this test, performed on 100 patients with complaints not related to the blood, will reveal several who would benefit from antianemia therapy. Hemoglobin, serology and urinalysis examinations are performed routinely on most patients. Many physicians and hospitals also include a blood count, test of the feces for blood, chest x-ray, and an electrocardiogram.

Some tests have no significance other than to indicate the diagnosis. An example of this is the glucose tolerance test. Should the result of such a test indicate the presence of diabetes, the test is of no further use in regulating treatment. Many tests, however, can be useful in following the course of the disease or in adjusting therapy. An example of the latter is the test for prothrombin time. In treatment with Dicumarol and similar drugs, tests for prothrombin time are performed daily to aid in prescribing the correct dose of Dicumarol for the current day.

In some institutions a single laboratory performs all the tests; in others there may be several laboratories, one performing bacteriological tests, another chemical tests, and so on.

The origin of the test material does not always correspond to the organ or system being examined. A test may be performed on urine to obtain information on liver function. Since, in the following chapters, the tests are arranged according to the type of specimen examined (i.e., blood, urine, etc.), tables 1-9 are included as a supplement which groups the tests according to the organ or system whose functions are being tested.

It should be noted that many of the tests are useful in diagnosing diseases of more than one organ or system. This, of course, is a natural consequence of the interrelationship between the various organs and systems of the body. In many cases, therefore, the interpretation of the results of these tests by the physician is not simply a matter of routine but involves careful integration with history and physical findings.

In some cases the relationship of a laboratory test to the pathological physiology of a disease is clear. For example, since the kidney excretes urea, it might be predicted that in advanced kidney disease the blood urea levels will be elevated. On the other hand, the exact relationship of some laboratory tests to the pathological physiology of disease is not known. An example of this is the thymol turbidity test for liver function. In these cases it has been found empirically that the tests are usually positive in certain types of disorders. There are theories which attempt to correlate the test results with the disease process, but since they are unproven, and in most cases highly complex, they are not discussed in this book.

There are other tests, such as the determination of the sedimentation rate, which are so non-specific that they do not point to any particular group of diseases, but only indicate that there is some disorder.

Drugs. In evaluating laboratory tests, it is always advisable to consider the drugs which a patient is receiving. In a number of cases, these drugs can affect the test results and produce an erroneous diagnosis. As more and more drugs are developed, this problem will increase in complexity. New drugs are being developed so rapidly at present that even an up-to-date book may not be a complete enough guide to the ways in which drugs can interfere with laboratory tests. Furthermore, the physician in charge of the patient is seldom aware of technical details of laboratory procedures and the ways in which drugs can interfere with them. On the other hand, the clinical pathologist in charge of the laboratory who does have this information may not know which drugs have been administered to the patient. The nurse is in a position to help in the solution of this problem. In most hospitals, the laboratory slip which is sent from the ward to the laboratory along with the specimen has a space for a brief clinical summary or impression. It is suggested that the nurse include therein a list of all the drugs which the patient has received in the past 72 hours. Perhaps, in the future, these laboratory slips will include a special space for listing all drugs being administered to the patient.

In the discussion of each test in this book, a special section lists the known drugs, foods and procedures which have been reported to interfere with or give erroneous results in laboratory tests. Although every effort has been made to include all published information on interference with laboratory test results, it must be assumed that the information listed is incomplete.

We do not know in every case if the drugs listed are likely to interfere with a test occasionally, usually, or all the time. Accordingly, it may be quite proper for a physician to order a laboratory test even though he knows that a potentially interfering drug is being administered, provided his interpretation of the results considers the possible effects of interference. On the other hand, it is certainly preferable to do the tests in the absence of potentially interfering materials.

There are several mechanisms whereby laboratory results may be changed by interfering materials. In some cases, there is an effect on the laboratory procedure, producing an incorrect measurement. For example, the test for bilirubin is based on the color of the serum. If the patient has taken a drug or a food which gives a yellowish color to the serum, the test reading will be high, even though the actual bilirubin level may be normal.

In other cases, a food, medication, or test material may contribute increased amounts of a particular substance to body fluids. The actual test reading may be perfectly correct and accurate, but it may still be misleading if the role of the additional substance is not recognized. For example, in possible cases of hypothyroidism, a low protein-bound iodine is an important diagnostic point. Many drugs (table 22), including over-the-counter remedies, contain iodine, and may produce an elevation of the protein-bound iodine. If a patient has taken one of these drugs and has an elevated protein-bound iodine level as a result, the physician may be misled in his diagnosis unless he is aware of the possible effects of the drug on the test results.

In other situations, drugs may confuse the diagnosis because of mild to moderate toxic effects on some organs. If a patient has obscure symptoms which the physician is trying to diagnose, several tests of liver function may be ordered, such as transaminase levels (SGOT). Many drugs can elevate SGOT levels, probably because of slight liver toxicity. If the patient has taken one of these drugs, and the physician is not aware of it, or of the possible relationship to test results, he could mistakenly conclude that the probable diagnosis was early liver disease when, in actuality, an entirely different condition might be involved.

It must be borne in mind that the information in this book is a summary of the available knowledge of the subject. The descriptions of the laboratory tests themselves are abbreviated as much as possible. A laboratory test described in 2 or 3 lines here might require 2 or 3 pages of description in order to enable the reader to understand it fully and to perform it. For a thorough understanding of the laboratory procedures, a standard book on laboratory methods should be consulted.

The vast majority of clinical cases in which laboratory tests aid in diagnosis will be covered by the tests in this book.

However, in some cases in which the diagnosis is still obscure after the usual test results are available, the physician may need a group of tests or some additional, less common tests. This occurs mainly with the liver diseases and with some chronic disorders of connective tissue. On the basis of clinical experience, tables have been devised which help the physician (usually a consultant) use a series of test results to arrive at a correct diagnosis of an obscure ailment. Material of this sort is beyond the scope of this book, and the reader who wishes to have such information is directed to the more comprehensive texts and the original clinical studies.

As additional aids Chapters 8, 9, 10 and tables 10-27 are included.

Chapter 8 summarizes the important distinctions to be made between normal values for adults, and for infants and children.

Chapter 9 consists of a description of the units of measurement used in clinical laboratory procedures.

Chapter 10 summarizes the principal rules that apply to the technique of venipuncture.

The tables 10-15 are designed for quick reference for the nurse on duty who needs to know how much blood or other material is required for a particular test, whether anticoagulant is added, and what type of container is to be used. Normal ranges for adults are included in these tables.

Tables 16 through 27 list drugs in various pharmacologic groups which may interfere with laboratory test results.

PART ONE

2

Bacteriological Tests

Materials collected for bacteriological examination fall into two groups: (1) cultures made at the bedside, and (2) specimens to be cultured in the laboratory.

A *culture* consists of material inoculated directly into a culture medium. In most hospitals only nose and throat secretions and venous blood are put into culture media at the bedside. The culture should be placed in an incubator at once, so that the bacteria may grow.

A *specimen* consists of material which will be cultured in the laboratory. All bacteriological specimens, other than spinal fluid, are kept in the bacteriological refrigerator to preserve the organisms. Spinal fluid may contain organisms which are sensitive to cold and is therefore placed in a bacteriological incubator.

In handling specimens and cultures for bacteriological examinations, it is at all times essential to keep in mind the possible danger of spreading infectious agents. All persons handling bacteriological material must know the necessary protective procedures. It is also important that the specimens reach the laboratory in a condition suitable for culture. Accordingly, the following precautions must be observed:

1. Use standard equipment. Do not substitute other containers for those designated by the laboratory.
2. Do not use cracked or broken containers.
3. Use only the regulation plugs to stopper tubes and bottles. Do not substitute gauze, paper, ordinary cotton, or other materials.
4. Do not use applicators which are broken or in any way contaminated.

5. Use only one applicator per tube.
6. Do not use Petri dishes for specimens which are fluid or which ooze fluids, including blood, except in bedside blood cultures.
7. Remove plugs from containers gently, with a twisting motion; do not pull straight out.
8. Discard any plug which comes in contact with an unsterile surface.
9. No not fill containers more than half-full.
10. Do not allow plugs to become wet, either from the specimen or from other sources. Wet plugs may contaminate personnel handling them and may also contaminate the specimen.
11. Do not spill any material on the outside of containers, plugs, boxes, tables, etc. If such material is spilled accidentally, call the bacteriology laboratory to find out how best to destroy the infectious agent. Ordinary soap and water may not be adequate. Do not allow anyone to come near the spilled material.
12. Make sure that plugs are firmly in place when the procedure is completed.
13. Plugs should be rotated clockwise.
14. Specimens and cultures should be carried in an upright position, and should not be shaken.
15. After collection, the specimen should be sent to the laboratory at once.
16. Certain organisms such as the gonococcus and the Pertussis and Brucella groups need freshly prepared culture media. Therefore, if the presence of those organisms is suspected, the laboratory must be notified at least an hour before the specimen is collected.

Agglutination Tests

The blood is tested for substances made by the body to neutralize a particular invading organism. These substances, known as agglutinins, cause such microorganisms to clump together. When specific agglutinins are present, they indicate that the body has been exposed to the microorganism in question and has developed some immunity to it. This procedure can be used with a large variety of microorganisms. However, only three groups are usually tested for in most laboratories in this country. They are:

1. The Brucella, or undulant fever, group of bacteria.
2. The typhoid and paratyphoid group of bacteria. The Widal test is used.
3. Rickettsia. This agglutination reaction differs from the others in that the organism which is agglutinated is not the rickettsia itself but a bacterium, Proteus OX19, which for some unknown reason is agglutinated by the anti-rickettsial agglutinins. The test used is also known as the Weil-Felix test.

There is an important consideration in judging the results of these tests. A positive test indicates only that the patient harbored the microorganism *at some time;* it does not necessarily indicate that the organism is still present. A patient who had the suspected disease years previously may still have a positive agglutination reaction.

Food and Drink Restrictions. None.

Procedure for Collecting Specimen. 5 ml. of venous blood is placed in a test tube and allowed to coagulate. The tests are performed on the serum. The quantity is sufficient for all three agglutination tests. Particular care must be exercised to prevent the spilling of blood on the outside of the test tube since blood may contain virulent organisms.

Laboratory Procedure. The laboratory adds serial dilutions of the patient's serum to suspensions of either live or killed bacteria. Observations are then made, sometimes with and sometimes without a microscope, to see whether clumping has occurred and to determine the range of dilutions within which the agglutination takes place. The dilutions ordinarily used range up to 1:1024. When live bacteria are used, they remain virulent when agglutinated and must be disposed of carefully.

Possible Interfering Materials and Conditions. If the patient has received antibiotics or chemotherapy (such as sulfonamides) there may be a false negative report.

Normal Range. Normal people sometimes have small amounts of agglutinin in their blood. Accordingly, the lowest concentration of the serum at which agglutination takes place is important. In the Widal test for typhoid fever, a positive agglutination at a concentration of 1:160 and up is required for a definite diagnosis. Separate measurements of 0, H, and V, antigens may be made.

In the diagnosis of brucellosis by agglutination, a positive response at serum dilution of 1:50 or over is required, depending on the skin test.

In the Weil-Felix test for rickettsial disease, agglutination must take place at serum dilutions of 1:160 or more for the test to be positive.

If there is doubt as to whether a positive agglutination test comes from a current infection or an earlier one, repeated tests may be performed at intervals of 3 to 5 days. Agglutination in progressively higher dilutions of serum strongly suggests a current infection.

Antibiotic Sensitivity Test

It is sometimes important to know which antibiotic is most effective against a particular strain of bacteria causing a patient's illness. This can sometimes be determined in the laboratory, using the disc or tube dilution methods. Since there are many variables which determine the effectiveness of antibiotics, these tests are only suggestive.

Food and Drink Restrictions. None.

Procedure for Collecting Specimen. The same as for corresponding cultures.

If both antibiotic sensitivity and blood culture tests are ordered together, it may be possible to do both on the blood culture material. However, this will vary according to the system used in a particular laboratory, and the laboratory should be consulted first.

Laboratory Procedure. The ability of various antibiotics to stop or slow the multiplication of bacteria is measured. There are several methods which may be used. The most common of these is the disc method which involves placing small discs of filter paper containing an antibiotic on a Petri dish streaked with a culture of the bacteria. The width of the zone of growth inhibition around the disc determines the sensitivity of the organism to the antibiotic. In the tube dilution method, the bacteria are cultured in a series of tubes containing known concentrations of an antibiotic. The lowest concentration completely inhibiting multiplication of the bacteria determines the sensitivity of the organism.

Possible Interfering Materials and Conditions. If the patient has received antibiotic or chemotherapy (such as sulfonamides) there may be a false negative report.

Blood Culture

Many varieties of bacteria may produce bacteremia or bloodstream infections. Frequently, a precise identification of the offending microorganism is necessary to enable the physician to select the appropriate antibiotic. Some types of bacteria do not survive changes in temperature or prolonged standing in the absence of special culture media, so that it is impractical to send a specimen of venous blood to be cultured. The procedure, therefore, is carried out at the bedside.

Food and Drink Restrictions. None.

Procedure for Collecting Specimen. There are several different procedures available.

Newer Method. The patient's skin must be properly prepared with an effective antiseptic. Either benzalkonium chloride or iodine followed by alcohol may be used. Newer methods of obtaining blood cultures are based on the use of prepared blood culture media in special vacuum bottles, and special blood-taking units. The procedure is simplified since it is merely necessary to insert one needle of the blood-taking unit into the patient's vein, and the other needle into the vacuum bottle. When the appropriate amount of blood has poured into the bottle, the tubing is clamped, the needle removed from the vacuum bottle, and then the other needle removed from the patient's vein. The bottle is then labelled and sent to the laboratory for further procedures.

The precautions necessary to prevent contamination of the culture are just as important as with the older method.

Older Method.

Materials. A blood culture set usually consists of the following:

    a. Two Petri dishes.
    b. One bottle of infusion broth with glucose.
    c. One bottle of plain infusion broth, which may have penicillinase added if the patient has received penicillin.
    d. Two tubes of agar.

The following steps are taken:

1. The stoppered tubes of agar are heated in a container of boiling water until the material is completely liquefied.
2. Place the tubes of agar in a container of water 50° C *as measured with a thermometer.* If the temperature falls below 45° C the agar will solidify and have to be remelted. If the temperature is above 50° C the bacteria may be destroyed.
3. Prepare the patient's skin at the site of venipuncture with a suitable antiseptic (tinctures of iodine or benzalkonium chloride) and draw 13 cc. of blood into a sterile syringe.
4. Place 5 cc. of blood in each bottle of broth.
5. Place 1 cc. of blood in one Petri dish and 2 cc. in the other.
6. Add the agar at 50° C to the blood and cover the Petri dishes. Rotate gently, without splashing, to mix uniformly.
7. Allow the agar in the Petri dish to solidify for *at least*

10 minutes. Then invert and place flat.

8. Label each container with name and location of patient, and *date* and *hour* when the culture was made.
9. Deliver the cultures to the laboratory or place them in the bacteriological incubator.

Laboratory Procedure. The laboratory will observe the cultures at regular intervals. If bacteriological growth appears, they will endeavor to identify the organism by direct smears. Frequently they will have to make one or more subcultures for positive identification. Final reports may therefore be delayed as long as 10 days. Usually, however, preliminary reports on blood cultures are available after 36 hours.

Possible Interfering Materials and Conditions. If the patient has received antibiotics or chemotherapy (such as sulfonamides) there may be a false negative report.

Normal Range. Normal blood should be sterile. Any microorganism found in the blood culture is either a contaminant from an imperfect procedure or indicates a pathological condition.

Dark-Field Examination

This is a variety of bacteriological examination which is usually done to determine whether the Treponema of syphilis is present. The test is performed on fluid oozing out of lesions of skin or mucous membranes, not on blood. This special type of examination is needed because the Treponema is too thin to be seen by ordinary microscopic techniques, but can be seen by reflected light in a dark field.

Food and Drink Restrictions. None.

Procedure for Collecting Specimen. The specimen is collected by the person (usually a bacteriologist or pathologist) doing the examination. In most institutions the patient is brought to the laboratory for this examination.

Precaution. Material from a dark-field positive lesion is highly infectious. All personnel who may come in contact with it should be protected.

Laboratory Procedure. The material is examined in a dark field for the Treponema pallidum. When an oral lesion is under examination, careful observation is needed to distinguish the Treponema pallidum from similar forms which are normally found in the mouth, and which do not cause disease.

Possible Interfering Materials and Conditions. If the patient has received antibiotics there may be a false negative report.

Normal Range. Normally there are no Treponema pallidum to be seen.

Fluorescent Antibody

This is a rapid test for the identification of microorganisms. It is usually used to determine the type of organism involved in an infection so that the most appropriate antibiotic can be chosen at once. This procedure also can be used to identify particular microorganisms in a mixture of many types. It can identify bacteria, protozoa, viruses and proteins. In medicolegal applications, a similar technique can be used to identify the species origin of minute blood stains. In epidemiological studies, a similar technique can determine the species of animal upon which a mosquito has last fed. There are also Civil Defense aspects to this test. Since it can identify organisms within a matter of minutes, it could be used in suspected biological warfare attacks to determine which organisms are being spread.

A recent development is the fluorescent treponemal antibody test. In this test, the ability of a patient's serum to coat treponemes is measured. Although this is probably the most specific and sensitive of all the serologic tests for syphilis, it requires special techniques and training and is not yet performed in most hospitals. However, if advisable, the patient's serum may be sent for testing to an institution which does perform this procedure.

Food and Drink Restrictions. None.

Procedure for Collecting Specimen. Specimens are collected in a sterile, clean disposable container, and sent to the laboratory at once. This test may be done on almost any type of body fluid. It is advisable to indicate to the laboratory which microorganisms are suspected.

Laboratory Procedure. Specific antisera, conjugated with a fluorescent material (fluorescein isothiocyanate) which may be obtained from several commercial sources are used. The specimen to be examined is fixed to a slide and fluorescent antiserum layered over it. After a few minutes, the excess antiserum is washed off, and the slide examined by ultraviolet light in a special microscope. If any of the fluorescein remains, it will glow in the ultraviolet light. When the test is properly performed, the fluorescence will be seen only where the antibody has combined with the proper antigen. For example, if it is suspected that there are typhoid bacilli in a specimen, the laboratory will place fluorescein conjugated antityphoid antiserum on the slide. After washing, the antityphoid antiserum would remain and fluoresce only if typhoid bacilli were present in the specimen.

Possible Interfering Materials and Conditions. If the patient has received antibiotics or chemotherapy (such as sulfonamides) there may be a false negative report.

Normal Range. This depends on the type of specimen being examined.

Fluorescent Treponemal Antibody Absorption (FTA-ABS)

This is a test for syphilis, the most sensitive currently known. It is used when other tests suggest syphilis, but when a false positive reaction must be ruled out.

Food and Drink Restrictions. None reported.

Procedure for Collecting Specimen. Venous blood is withdrawn and 5 cc. placed in a test tube and allowed to coagulate. The test is performed on the serum.

Laboratory Procedure. The procedure is much more complex than that required for most serological tests for syphilis, and not all laboratories can perform it. In essence, the patient's serum is allowed to react with stored treponemes on a slide. Then, a fluorescein labeled anti-human globulin is added, and the slide examined with a fluorescent microscope.

Possible Interfering Materials and Conditions. In some cases of lupus erythematosus, a partial fluorescense consisting of a "beaded" pattern may be seen.

Normal Range. Normally, this test is negative.

Miscellaneous Fluid Cultures

Various body cavities sometimes fill with fluid which may contain bacteria. The pleural, peritoneal and pericardial cavities are most commonly involved.

Food and Drink Restrictions. None.

Procedure for Collecting Specimen. The physician removes the specimen and places it in a sterile tube, using aseptic technique.

Laboratory Procedure. Essentially the same as in blood culture test.

Possible Interfering Materials and Conditions. If the patient has received antibiotics or chemotherapy (such as sulfonamides) there may be a false negative report.

Normal Range. Normally these body cavities are sterile. Therefore, any bacteria found in the culture are either pathogenic or contaminants resulting from an imperfect collection procedure.

Nose and Throat Culture

It is frequently useful for the physician to know which bacteria are present in the nose and throat. This information is obtained by means of a nose and throat culture.

Food and Drink Restrictions. None.

Procedure for Collecting Specimen. The physician collects the specimen on a sterile cotton swab. The swab is suspended in a sterile culture tube containing 2 cc. of broth, *without touching the broth*. The broth is not a culture medium. It is used to keep the air around the swab moist so that evaporation and drying of the specimen do not occur. Special culture tubes containing Loeffler's medium are used when diphtheria is suspected. In the latter case, the medium does touch the swab.

In some institutions, culture tubes *without* any fluid are used. These are satisfactory if the specimens are taken to the laboratory without delay.

Laboratory Procedure. The swab is to be plated (streaked gently across a dish containing agar). The colonies that grow out will then be identified microscopically or, if necessary, subcultures will be made.

Possible Interfering Materials and Conditions. If the patient has received antibiotics or chemotherapy (such as sulfonamides) there may be a false negative report.

Normal Range. Many bacteria are normally found in the nose and throat, including pneumococci, staphylococci, streptococci, H. influenzae, K. pneumoniae, and others. The decision as to whether a particular type found in the culture is related to the patient's illness can usually be made only after the physician has correlated these and other findings. Certain types of bacteria, such as those causing tuberculosis or diphtheria, are always abnormal.

Spinal Fluid Culture

The spinal fluid is examined in cases of suspected meningitis. There are several kinds of microorganisms which may produce meningitis and precise identification is usually important in order that the most suitable antibiotic may be selected.

Food and Drink Restrictions. None.

Procedure for Collecting Specimen. The physician places 2 cc. of spinal fluid in a special small test tube. The specimen is stored in an incubator, not a refrigerator.

Laboratory Procedure. This is the same as in other cultures. Because of the urgency that exists in the case of meningitis, the laboratory will call the floor as soon as the organism has been identified.

Possible Interfering Materials and Conditions. If the patient has received antibiotics or chemotherapy (such as sulfonamides) there may be a false negative report.

Normal Range. The spinal fluid is normally sterile.

Sputum Culture

Sputum is material brought up from the lungs and trachea during deep coughing. It should not be confused with saliva or postnasal secretions. This test is often of value in diagnosing lung infections. Since sputum is often contaminated with postnasal secretions and saliva, the organisms found in these secretions may also occur in sputum cultures.

Food and Drink Restrictions. None.

Procedure for Collecting Specimen. The patient uses a special specimen cup or box with a cover. He is instructed to place the sputum raised by a few good coughs into the container. The container is delivered without delay to the bacteriology refrigerator. Containers holding sputum should not be allowed to remain at the bedside for hours. The patient must be warned not to get any sputum on the outside of the container, and it should never be completely filled. If the patient is in isolation, the outside of the container is contaminated and must be handled with the necessary technique to avoid spreading infection.

In some cases, 24-hour sputum specimens are ordered. In such cases, the containers should be replaced well before they are completely filled. Indeed, it may be prudent to leave an extra container with the patient.

Laboratory Procedure. Essentially the same as with other cultures with special attention to the presence of acid-fast (tubercle) bacilli.

Possible Interfering Materials and Conditions. If the patient has received antibiotics or chemotherapy (such as sulfonamides) there may be a false negative report.

Normal Range. Both pathogenic and nonpathogenic bac-

teria are found in some lung diseases. The physician, therefore, after correlating all his findings must decide whether a
particular finding is likely to be significant.

Stool Culture

The normal bacterial flora of the stool are the largest in
number and kind found in any part of the body. About 50
varieties of bacteria are normally present in the stool. There
are also several types of pathogenic bacteria. Different culture media are needed for some of the pathogenic bacteria.
The laboratory, therefore, should always be told which disease is suspected.

Food and Drink Restrictions. None.

Procedure for Collecting Specimen. Use special containers with properly fitted covers. Use a tongue depresor to
place a small amount of feces (about 1 inch in diameter) into
the container. Avoid contaminating the outside of the container. Deliver promptly to the bacteriology laboratory or
refrigerator. Specimens obtained at proctoscopy may be collected on swabs, as described in *Nose and Throat Culture.*

Laboratory Procedure. This will depend on the type of
pathogenic bacteria suspected.

Possible Interfering Materials and Conditions. If the patient has received antibiotics or chemotherapy (such as sulfonamides) there may be a false negative report.

Normal Range. About 50 types of bacteria are normally
present in the feces. Some not normally found may be harmless. Usually, specific pathogens such as those of typhoid, dys-
entery, brucellosis, etc., are sought for and reported if
present.

Tests for Special Microorganisms

Certain tests for virus and rickettsial disease are not ordinarily performed in the hospital laboratory but are sent to
a public health department laboratory. In large city health
departments or in state public health laboratories tests may

be performed for many diseases, including Colorado tick fever, influenza, mumps, psittacosis, Q-fever, typhus, and several kinds of virus encephalitis. Tests may also be performed for parasitic infestations such as amebiasis, trichinosis, and echinococcosis. Certain other diseases are tested for by the United States Public Health Laboratory, such as trypanosomiasis, schistosomiasis, filariasis, leishmaniasis, histoplasmosis, blastomycosis, toxoplasmosis, and leptospirosis.

Procedure for Collecting Specimen. Two specimens of blood are required. One is drawn during the acute phase of the disease and the other two weeks later. About 10 cc. of blood is placed in a test tube and allowed to coagulate. The specimen, needle and syringe are handled with great care to avoid contamination of personnel with infectious agents. Packing of the sample for shipment to the appropriate laboratory is done according to the directions of that laboratory. Special containers may usually be obtained from the hospital laboratory.

Treponemal Immobilization Test (TPI)

This is a highly specific test for syphilis with few, if any, false positives, but for technical reasons is very difficult to perform. It is being replaced by the fluorescent treponemal antibody absorption test.

Urine Culture

Urine culture is often of value in determining the etiological agent in infectious diseases of kidneys, ureters and bladder.

Food and Drink Restrictions. None.

Procedure for Collecting Specimen. In some cases it is possible to collect a sterile noncatheterized specimen from men after cleaning the genital area. However, even with all precautions, some contamination may occur. Therefore, noncatheterized specimens must be brought to the bacteriology laboratory at once, before the contaminating microorganisms multiply and crowd out the pathogens sought. For women patients it has been customary to use catheterized specimens only. However, recent studies have questioned this procedure. It has been shown that, despite all precautions, the insertion of a catheter into the bladder often introduces infection. *Accordingly, many doctors now believe that it is too risky to catheterize patients for urine culture.* Instead, a clean, voided specimen is used. The entire vulvar area is carefully cleansed, using benzalkonium (Zephiran). It should then be rinsed with sterile water. In place of benzalkonium, a hexachlorophene soap may be used followed by a sterile rinse. However, benzalkonium and hexachlorophene soap should not both be used. The labia are held apart and urine is voided into a sterile bottle. The urine culture is often contaminated by skin bacteria but contamination of the culture is preferable to contamination of the bladder. It is essential to note on the chart whether the urine specimen is passed normally or via catheter.

Laboratory Procedure. Essentially the same as in other types of culture.

Possible Interfering Materials and Conditions. If the patient has received antibiotics or chemotherapy (such as sulfonamides) there may be a false negative report.

Normal Range. Normal urine is sterile. Any bacteria found are contaminants from the skin, or invading organisms.

Weil-Felix Test

See Agglutination Tests

Widal Test

See Agglutination Tests

Wound Culture

When wounds or surgical incisions show evidence of infection, it is frequently important to identify the invading organism so that specific therapy may be instituted.

re it is the proper one, rather than to rely on the
f the stopper as a guide.

always advisable to draw enough blood into the va-
ube to fill it. This is particularly important when any
ated to blood clotting is to be performed, since inade-
lling of the tube may give spurious results. Unfortu-
some vacuum tubes that remain on the shelf for any
of time may lose part of their vacuum. Such tubes
be discarded at once.

t tests are designated as "routine." That is, they are
ed by the laboratory in the ordinary working sched-
ce there is no important medical advantage in having
lts available before late afternoon or the following
a few cases it may be necessary to know the results of
cular test as soon as possible. Such specimens are la-
emergency" and the test is carried out at once. The
ency" designation is the responsibility of the physician
ge and should be made only for genuine medical
It is improper to designate a test as an emergency in
o facilitate a patient's early discharge or because the
was drawn too late for routine testing that day.

en blood or other fluids known or suspected to be
ng a microorganism causing infectious disease are sent
er than bacteriological examination, the specimen
be labeled in red "Infectious Material." Examples are:
urine and stools from typhoid patients; spinal fluid in
itis; and blood in various rickettsial and virus diseases.

times a large number of blood determinations are
d for a patient on a single day. If the total amount of
eeded for all tests exceeds 20 cc., it may prove diffi-
impossible to obtain it from a particular patient,
larly one with poor circulation. Often, the labora-
manage to perform a satisfactory test with less blood
usually requested. Therefore, in the appropriate
t is advisable to call the laboratory in advance, and
ether they can perform the series of tests with less
than usual.

Food and Drink Restrictions. None.

Procedure for Collecting Specimen. The physician collects pus or exudate from the wound on a sterile cotton swab. The swab is placed in a sterile tube as described under *Nose and Throat Culture.*

Laboratory Procedure. The laboratory procedure is generally similar to other cultures. However, special efforts are made to culture anaerobic bacteria, since their presence is serious and requires special handling.

Possible Interfering Materials and Conditions. If the patient has received antibiotics or chemotherapy (such as sulfonamides) there may be a false negative report.

Normal Range. All wounds and surgical incisions are contaminated by bacteria. However, only a small proportion of them are actually infected. The significance of a culture, therefore, depends on the type of microorganism found and on the clinical picture. Normal skin flora include diphtheroids, E. coli, B. subtilis, P. vulgaris, streptococci, and staphylococci, but others are also found.

3

Tests Performed on Blood

Many test are performed on blood for diagnostic purposes. When only a drop or two of blood is needed for a test, such as a hemoglobin determination or white blood cell count, it is usually obtained by pricking the finger or ear lobe. This blood oozes from capillaries and is, therefore, called capillary blood. When a larger quantity is needed, it is obtained from a vein and is called venous blood.

Improper handling of the specimen may give erroneous and misleading results. It is thus essential that in collecting blood for the laboratory the following precautions be observed:

1. The patient should be in the fasting state for several tests. Absorption of food may alter many of the blood constituents. If fats are absorbed, their presence in the blood (lipemia) may interfere with some tests such as bilirubin, albumin-globulin ratio, and others.

2. Hemolysis will cause serious errors in many tests such as those for potassium serum bilirubin, and others. This can be avoided when a syringe is used by observing the following precautions:

   a. The syringe must be perfectly dry as well as sterile, since ordinary water will hemolyze red cells.

   b. When drawing the blood, an even pressure should be used in pulling back the plunger of the syringe. Avoid excessive negative pressure.

   c. After drawing the blood, remove the needle from the syringe and empty the latter into the correct container without foaming or splashing the blood.

   d. Do not use containers which have been chilled.

e. Avoid shaking the spec

3. Sometimes, a blood test is
is receiving intravenous i
tion is to take blood from
infusion. Nevertheless, th
ways be enough, since it
run on blood samples take
intravenous infusion going
been distorted. According
a patient while he is receiv
that fact should be noted
also on the slip sent to th

4. Concentration of the blo
should be prevented, or s
inaccurate results. In orde
quet should be removed fr
is definitely in the vein. All
while fresh venous blood f
blood into the syringe. Un
is ignored by many physic
some of the determinations
them are inaccurate. The
and only requires an addi

5. After specimens are drawn
laboratory as soon as poss
cannot be made at once, tl
for handling or treating the
stored safely.

There is increasing use of
tubes for drawing blood. These ha
tages over syringes. The vacuu
sizes, and with different typ
specific tests. They have rubber
but unfortunately, the manufac
same color stopper for different
it is important to check the actua

to be s
color o
It is
cuum t
test rel
quate f
nately,
length
should

Mos
perform
ule, sin
the res
day. In
a partic
beled "
"emerg
in cha
reasons
order t
sample
Wh
harbori
for oth
should
blood,
mening
At
ordered
blood
cult or
particu
tory ca
than i
cases,
ask wh
blood

A/G (Albumin-Globulin) Ratio

See Albumin, Globulin, Total Protein, A/G Ratio

Acid Phosphatase

See Phosphatase, Acid

Albumin, Globulin, Total Protein, A/G Ratio

These tests are usually performed together. They may be useful in the diagnosis of kidney, liver, and some other diseases.

The main function of the serum albumin appears to be the maintenance of osmotic pressure of the blood. The main function of serum globulin is not fully understood, but probably involves immunologic defense. One of its secondary functions is to assist in maintaining the osmotic pressure of the blood. Since the globulin molecule is several times as large as the albumin molecule it is less efficient, gram for gram, in maintaining osmotic pressure. In certain diseases the albumin may leak out of capillary walls, while the larger globulin molecules are retained within the blood stream. The body may then compensate for loss of albumin by producing more globulin, so that the globulin becomes responsible for a larger share of the osmotic pressure. Yet despite normal or even increased total dissolved protein in the serum, osmotic pressure may be less than normal because of the lesser effectiveness of globulin. As a result there may be some edema. By discovering a shift in the albumin-globulin ratio, the physician is aided in diagnosing the patient's illness. He may also rely on repeated albumin-globulin ratio determinations for judging the effectiveness of treatment.

Conditions in which the albumin-globulin ratio is lowered include chronic nephritis, lipoid nephrosis, liver disease, amyloid nephrosis, and malnutrition.

Food and Drink Restrictions. None.

Procedure for Collecting Specimen. Venous blood is withdrawn and 6 cc. placed in a test tube and allowed to coagulate. The test is performed on the serum.

Laboratory Procedure. The total protein in a sample of serum is determined by the Kjeldahl method. Then the albumin is separated from another sample of serum and the amount measured. The concentration of globulin is determined by subtracting the value for albumin from the total protein.

Possible Interfering Materials and Conditions. The level of serum proteins may be falsely elevated by Bromsulphalein (B.S.P.). Accordingly, the serum protein measurement should be delayed if the patient has had a B.S.P. test within the past 48 hours.

Normal Range:
Total serum protein, 6.0 to 8.0 Gm. per 100 cc. of serum;
Serum albumin, 3.2 to 5.6 Gm. per 100 cc. of serum;
Serum globulin, 1.3 to 3.2 Gm. per 100 cc. of serum;
A/G ratio, 1.5:1 to 2.5:1.

Alcohol

The concentration of blood alcohol in a patient may be needed for strictly medical or medicolegal purposes. If an unconscious or barely conscious patient is admitted to a hospital, one of the items to be considered in differential diagnosis is alcoholism. In other cases, the level of blood alcohol in a person who is definitely drunk may be helpful in determining the appropriate therapy. With moderate levels, the patient might just be allowed to sleep it off. However, if levels were dangerously high, more vigorous therapy might be indicated.

The medicolegal use of blood alcohol levels is usually based on laws relating to drunken driving. In most areas, Highway Patrol officers now use devices to measure alcohol concentration on the breath. This indirectly indicates blood levels. However, blood samples may be used in some cases, or a patient under arrest may request that his blood be tested as well as his breath.

Blood levels of alcohol under 0.05 % mean that the subject is not legally considered to be under the influence of

alcohol. However, physiologically, even such low levels reduce driving ability significantly. Levels between 0.05 % and
0.15 % may or may not be considered to mean that the subject is not legally considered to be under the influence of
evidence. Levels of 0.15 % and over are considered clear
evidence of being under the influence of alcohol. At levels
of 0.25 % and over, there is marked intoxication and beginning stupor. At about 0.40 %, coma occurs, and at slightly
higher levels, death can result.

Food and Drink Restrictions. None.

Procedure for Collecting Specimen. It is essential that no
alcohol be used for cleaning the patient's arm. Instead, a
solution of benzalkonium may be used to clean the venipuncture area, and then wiped off gently with a sterile swab or
sponge. However, a *tincture* must not be used, since it contains alcohol.

Venous blood is withdrawn, and 10 ml. placed in a test
tube and allowed to coagulate. The test is performed on the ,
serum, but it can also be performed on whole blood which
has been treated with an anticoagulant.

Laboratory Procedure. The sample is subjected to a diffu-
sion or distillation technique to separate the alcohol from
the serum or blood. The diffusate or distillate is then added
to an acid dichromate solution, producing a color change
which can be measured by colorimetry or titration.

Possible Interfering Materials and Conditions. Methyl
alcohol (wood alcohol) and isopropyl alcohol can produce
measurable levels.

Normal Range. Normally there is no alcohol in the blood.

Alkaline Phosphatase

See Phosphatase, Alkaline

Ammonia

This is primarily a test of liver function. Ammonia is
usually produced by bacterial action in the intestine and

absorbed into the blood. The liver ordinarily converts the ammonia into urea which is excreted by the kidneys. When the liver is diseased, its ability to convert ammonia to urea diminishes, and the blood ammonia level rises.

Other conditions which interfere temporarily with liver function may also cause a rise in blood ammonia levels. These include: congestive heart failure, shock, diabetic coma, and severe pneumonia. A change in the vascular pattern such as a portacaval shunt which permits venous blood from the intestines to bypass the liver and enter the general circulation could also increase blood ammonia levels.

Food and Drink Restrictions. None.

Procedure for Collecting Specimen. Notify the laboratory in advance so that they can be prepared to do the test without delay. Venous blood is withdrawn, and 5 ml. placed in a tube containing an appropriate anticoagulant. The acceptable anticoagulants are potassium oxalate, EDTA and some brands of heparin.

Laboratory Procedure. There are several procedures in use. One involves diffusing the ammonia into special bottles, and adding Nessler reagent. The result is read by photometer.

Possible Interfering Materials and Conditions. The serum ammonia level may be spuriously elevated by the following drugs (asterisk indicates the official or the common name):

°Acetazolamide	°Heparin (some brands)
°Ammonium salts	°Ion exchange resins (some)
°Chlorothiazide	°Methicillin
Diamox	Staphcillin
Dimocillin	°Thiazide drugs
Diuril	°Urea

Normal Range. The normal range depends on the techniques and experience of the laboratory doing the test, since many factors in the laboratory procedures and timing can influence results. Authoritative sources place the normal range at less than 75 micrograms per 100 cc. of blood.

Amylase

In certain types of pancreatic disease, the digestive enzymes of the pancreas escape into the surrounding tissue, producing necrosis with severe pain and inflammation. Under these circumstances there is an increase in the serum amylase. A serum amylase level of twice normal usually indicates acute pancreatitis. However, there are times when the serum amylase is elevated in abdominal conditions, such as intestinal obstruction. In mumps and other diseases of the salivary glands or ducts, the serum amylase reaches high levels, equivalent to those found in acute pancreatitis.

Some surgeons order routine serum amylase tests for the first few days after any operation which might have injured the pancreas. Whenever an elevation in the amylase level is found, they can institute therapy for pancreatitis early, thus increasing the patient's chances for recovery.

This test remains positive for a short time only, seldom for more than a few days.

Food and Drink Restrictions. None.

Procedure for Collecting Specimen. Venous blood is withdrawn and a 6 cc. sample allowed to coagulate in a test tube. At times this test may be designated "emergency" by the physician.

Laboratory Procedure. Starch in solution is hydrolyzed by the serum amylase. The amount of reducing sugar present is measured before and after the hydrolysis, and the difference indicates the serum amylase activity.

Possible Interfering Materials and Conditions. Even tiny droplets of saliva contaminating the specimen can cause spurious elevations of amylase readings since saliva has a high concentration of amylase. Therefore, improper pipetting, coughing, sneezing and, when the specimen is in an open container, sometimes even talking near it, either in the patient's room or the laboratory, can result in a misleading report.

The amylase levels may be elevated into distinctly abnormal levels if the patient has received any of the following drugs within 24 hours of drawing the blood sample (asterisk indicates the official or the common name):

*Bethanechol
*Codeine
Demerol
Diatrizoate, sodium
*Ethyl alcohol (large amounts)
Hypaque
Indocin
*Indomethacin
*Meperidine
*Methyl alcohol (large amounts
*Methylcholine
*Morphine
*Narcotic drugs
*Pentazocine
Talwin
Urecholine

The elevation of serum amylase levels which occurs after the administration of codeine, meperidine (Demerol) or morphine apparently depends on the pancreas being in a state of active secretion when the drugs are given. Therefore, if the patient has not had any food for at least four hours before administration of one of these narcotic drugs, an elevated serum amylase level can often be interpreted in the same manner as if a narcotic drug had not been given.

An extremely rare condition, macroamylasemia may produce elevated serum amylase levels without apparent pancreatitis.

Normal Range. 80 to 150 units (Somogyi).

Antiglobulin

See Coombs' Direct

Anti-Streptolysin O Titer

This test, usually used in suspected rheumatic fever, indicates the reaction of the body to a recent streptococcal infection. The streptococcus produces many enzymes, one of which, streptolysin O, has the ability to destroy red blood corpuscles. Part of the defense against this bacterium is an antibody which neutralizes streptolysin. Since rheumatic fever is related to a recent streptococcal infection, an increase in the titer of the anti-streptolysin is usually found in rheumatic fever. It should be clear, however, that this test, like all others useful in rheumatic fever, is nonspecific and can be positive in many other conditions.

Infants and young children sometimes have normal anti-streptolysin titers despite clear-cut rheumatic fever.

Food and Drink Restrictions. None.

Procedure for Collecting Specimen. Venous blood is withdrawn and 5 cc. placed in a test tube and allowed to clot. The test is performed on the serum.

Laboratory Procedure. A purified streptolysin from a streptococcus culture is standardized for its ability to dissolve rabbit red blood cells in suspension. Serial dilutions of the patient's serum are then tested to determine the greatest dilution which will prevent this effect of streptolysin.

Possible Interfering Materials and Conditions. None reported yet.

Normal Range. Up to 166 Todd units per cc. of serum.

Ascorbic Acid (Vitamin C)

This test is being performed much less often now than in the past, but it remains an important diagnostic tool. Ascorbic acid is an essential vitamin found in fresh fruits and vegetables. Deficiences are not uncommon, and may even occur in persons on an apparently adequate diet, who are taking vitamin supplements. The severe deficiency, scurvy, is rare and is usually readily recognized. However, relative deficiencies may occur in several conditions, and interfere with recovery. For example, in patients with severe burns, the need for ascorbic acid is markedly increased. The same may be true of those with severe infections. In some cancer patients, through mechanisms that are not clear, the ascorbic acid level may be quite low despite an adequate diet and presumably therapeutic supplements of the vitamin. This fact may be important, since ascorbic acid is vital to the body's defense mechanisms. For all of these reasons, it is often helpful to know the patient's ascorbic acid level.

Food and Drink Restrictions. None.

Procedure for Collecting Specimen. Venous blood is withdrawn and a 6 cc. sample placed in an oxalate bottle or tube. Another acceptable anticoagulant is heparin. The test is performed on plasma pipetted from the sample.

Laboratory Procedure. Several different methods are available. Most of them are based on the ability of ascorbic acid to decolorize a solution made blue by the addition of a special reagent.

Possible Interfering Materials and Conditions. None reported yet.

Normal Range. 0.6 to 1.6 mg. per 100 cc. of blood plasma.

Ascorbic Acid (Vitamin C) Tolerance (Blood)

See also Ascorbic Acid Tolerance (Urine)

This test measures the degree of ascorbic acid deficiency. Although it is not as widely performed as before, it can provide important clinical information since some persons with seemingly adequate diets, and even some receiving supplemental vitamins, may have a partial deficiency of ascorbic acid. This may be true of patients with severe burns, infection, or malignancy. A partial deficiency of ascorbic acid can interfere with wound healing, body defenses, and recovery.

Food and Drink Restrictions. For 24 hours before the test, the patient must avoid foods high in ascorbic acid. Water may be taken as desired.

Procedure for Collecting Specimen. The physician administers 10 mg./kg. of ascorbic acid as a 4% solution in sterile saline intravenously. Four hours after the injection, venous blood is withdrawn, and 6 cc. placed in an oxalate bottle or tube. Another acceptable anticoagulant is heparin. The test is performed on plasma and may be performed in conjunction with the urine test (P. 140).

Laboratory Procedure. The amount of ascorbic acid is measured photometrically after chemical modification.

Possible Interfering Materials and Conditions. None reported yet.

Normal Range. 1.5 mg./100 ml. or higher.

Australia Antigen

See Hepatitis Test

Bacillus Subtilis Inhibition

See Guthrie

Barbiturate

Barbiturate levels in the serum of unconscious patients are measured when there is a possibility of accidental or suicidal ingestion of an overdose of barbiturate. If high levels are found, therapy can be directed in a more meaningful way at the cause of the unconsciousness. The evaluation of the significance of high barbiturate levels is complicated by several factors. Other drugs including tranquilizers and alcohol can intensify the effects of moderate levels of barbiturates. Furthermore, the available tests do not yet permit the doctor to tell exactly which barbiturate has been ingested, and different barbiturates produce coma at different blood levels. The long-acting barbiturates such as phenobarbital (Luminal) produce coma at blood levels of about 8 mgm. per 100 cc. The medium-duration barbiturates such as amobarbital (Amytal) require levels of about 4 mgm. per 100 cc., and the short-acting barbiturates such as secobarbital (Seconal) and pentobarbital (Nembutal) only require levels of about 2 to 2.5 mgm. per 100 cc. to produce coma. Measurement of blood barbiturate level is almost always done on an emergency basis.

Food and Drink Restrictions. None.

Procedure for Collecting Specimen. Venous blood is withdrawn and 5 ml. placed in a test tube and allowed to coagulate.

Laboratory Procedure. The serum is extracted with chloroform, and alkali added to the extract. Differential ultraviolet spectrophotometry is then used to measure barbiturate concentration.

Possible Interfering Materials and Conditions. The barbiturate level may be spuriously elevated by the following:

Antipyrine
Theophylline (large doses)

Normal Range. Normally, there are no barbiturates in the blood.

Bilirubin, Partition (Direct and Indirect van den Bergh Test)

When the ability of the liver to excrete bilirubin is impaired by obstruction, either within or outside the organ, it is believed that the excess circulating bilirubin is free of any attached protein. However, when the increase in circulating bilirubin is due to increased destruction of red blood cells (hemolysis), it is believed that the bilirubin is bound to protein. By measuring the amount of free bilirubin (direct) and the amount bound to protein (indirect), there is some indication as to whether the patients's illness is based on obstruction or hemolysis.

Food and Drink Restrictions. None.

Procedure for Collecting Specimen. Venous blood is withdrawn and 5 cc. placed in a test tube and allowed to coagulate. The test is performed on the serum, but it is also possible to use plasma separated from uncoagulated blood.

Laboratory Procedure. The direct method is described below. In the indirect method alcohol is added to the sample of serum. The serum proteins precipitate, freeing any bilirubin which was bound to them, and the bilirubin dissolves in the alcohol. Ehrlich's reagent is then added to the alcoholic extract and the intensity of the color produced is measured.

Possible Interfering Materials and Conditions. The serum bilirubin may be spuriously high if the patient has had foods or drugs that impart an orange or yellow color to the serum. There may also be elevated levels when the patient has taken drugs that temporarily modify liver function. In such cases, the elevated levels may be real rather than spurious, but they do not indicate liver disease. The materials in both categories are listed below, by official (generic) name only, because of the large number involved:

Acetohexamide	Oxacillin
Anabolic agents, some	Phenothiazines
Androgens, some	Phytonadione
Aspidium	Pipobroman
Carotene	Pyrazinamide
Carrots	Quinacrine
Chlordiazepoxide	Radiopaque contrast media,
Erythromycin	some
Indomethacin	Salicylates (large amounts)
Isoniazid	Sulfonamides
Lipochrome	Triacetyloleandomycin
Menadiol (large amounts)	Trifluperidol
Mercaptopurine	Vitamin A
Methanol	Vitamin K in large doses in
Nitrofurantoin	newborn
Novobiocin	

Normal Range. 0.1 to 1.0 mg. per 100 cc. Within the normal range there is no significance to the ratio between the amounts of bilirubin found on direct and indirect measurements. When the concentration of bilirubin rises significantly over 1.0 mg. per 100 cc. the relative amounts which are free and bound to protein may suggest the type of disorder. If most of the bilirubin is found on the direct test, the chances are that the patient has an obstructive lesion. If most of it is found on the indirect test, the illness is likely to be hemolytic. These interpretations indicate probabilities, not certainties, and there is some controversy about the meaning of these tests.

Bilirubin, Total

Bilirubin is derived from the hemoglobin in red blood cells which have been broken down. It is constantly being produced, and is excreted by the liver into the bile, of which it is the chief pigment. There is always a small amount in the serum. When the destruction of red blood cells becomes excessive or when the liver is unable to excrete the ordinary quantities of bilirubin produced, the concentration in the serum rises. If the concentration becomes very high, there is visible jaundice. It is advantageous to discover the increased concentration of serum bilirubin before jaundice is seen, and that is accomplished by this test.

Food and Drink Restrictions. None.

Procedure for Collecting Specimen. Venous blood is withdrawn and 5 cc. placed in a test tube and allowed to coagulate. The test is performed on the serum but it is also possible to use plasma separated from uncoagulated blood.

Laboratory Procedure. To the sample of serum is added Ehrlich's reagent. A colored product is formed and the intensity of the color is used as a measure of the bilirubin concentration.

Possible Interfering Materials and Conditions. The serum bilirubin may be spuriously high if the patient has had foods or drugs that impart an orange or yellow color to the serum. There may also be elevated levels when the patient has taken drugs that temporarily modify liver function. In such cases, the elevated levels may be real rather than spurious, but they do not indicate liver disease. The materials in both categories are listed below, by official (generic) name only, because of the large number involved:

Acetohexamide   Androgens, some
Anabolic agents, some   Aspidium

Carotene
Carrots
Chlordiazepoxide
Erythromycin
Indomethacin
Isoniazid
Lipochrome
Menadiol (large amounts)
Mercaptopurine
Methanol
Nitrofurantoin
Novobiocin
Oxacillin
Phenothiazines

Phytonadione
Pipobroman
Pyrazinamide
Quinacrine
Radiopaque contrast
    media, some
Salicylates (large
    amounts)
Sulfonamides
Triacetyloleandomycin
Trifluperidol
Vitamin A
Vitamin K in large doses
    in newborn

Normal Range. 0.1 to 1.0 mg. per 100 cc. of serum.

Bleeding Time

This test measures the time during which there is bleeding from a small skin incision. It is quite distinct from tests. for clotting time and gives somewhat different information since, in a bleeding time test, constriction of the small vessels is also involved. Bleeding time is prolonged in thrombocytopenic purpura and other blood disorders.

Food and Drink Restrictions. None.

Procedure for Performing Test and Collecting Specimen. A standardized puncture wound of the skin is produced with an appropriate instrument. The site of the puncture may be the finger tip, ear lobe, or forearm. In some variations when the arm is used, a blood pressure cuff increases the venous pressure to make the test more sensitive. After the puncture is produced, the drops of blood are wiped away with filter paper every 30 seconds. The time at which bleeding stops is recorded.

Possible Interfering Materials and Conditions. None reported yet.

Normal Range. 1 to 6 minutes.

Blood Counts

Frequently, various blood cell and platelet counts are ordered either routinely to help with a particular problem, or to follow the results of treatment. Several counts are often performed together and will, therefore, be considered together here. Blood counts are performed on whole blood, usually capillary blood, although venous blood can be used.

Although the procedures described here are basic and still in wide use, they are rapidly being supplanted by electronic counters in most large institutions.

Complete blood count (CBC) refers to red cell count, white cell count, and white cell differential count.

Platelet Count

The platelets (thrombocytes), which are necessary for the clotting of blood, are particles much smaller than red blood cells. They are reduced in such conditions as thrombocytopenic purpura, aplastic anemia, Goucher's disease, and septicemia. They may be increased in polycythemia, fractures, and certain kinds of anemia.

Food and Drink Restrictions. None.

Procedure for Performing Test and Collecting Specimen. The procedure is essentially the same as for red blood cell counts, but employs a special diluting fluid.

Possible Interfering Materials and Conditions. None reported yet.

Normal Range. 200,000 to 500,000 per cubic mm.

Red Cell Count

The red cells (erythrocytes) contain hemoglobin, the essential oxygen carrier of the blood. An increase in red cells may indicate hemoconcentration (insufficient water in the blood), or polycythemia, which is a condition characterized by a persistently elevated red cell count. A reduction in the red cells may come from hemorrhage or one of the anemias.

Food and Drink Restrictions. None.

Procedure for Performing Test and Collecting Specimen. In the older method, the finger or ear lobe is punctured and blood drawn into a special red cell pipette, up to a given mark. Diluting solution is then added to a second mark and the contents thoroughly mixed. The diluted suspension is then allowed to flow into a space in a special counting chamber. Through the use of a microscope, the cells per unit area are then counted and the number of cells calculated. Newer methods use electronic counters.

Possible Interfering Materials and Conditions. None reported yet.

Normal Range. 4,000,000 to 6,000,000 per cubic mm. (Note that the unit of volume used, a cubic mm., is only 1/1,000 of a cc.)

Reticulocyte Count

This test gives some indication of bone marrow activity. Reticulocytes are immature red blood cells. They retain a network of reticular material which can be stained with the proper dyes. When the bone marrow cells are very active, (a situation which occurs after hemorrhage and with recovery from anemia), there is an increase in the number of reticulocytes in the blood. When the bone marrow cells are less active, the number of reticulocytes in the blood falls.

This test is often performed to evaluate the response to anemia therapy.

Food and Drink Restrictions. None.

Procedure for Performing Test and Collecting Specimen. A thin film of cresyl blue is allowed to dry on a glass slide. A fresh drop of blood is then spread over the stain and kept moist to allow the stain to penetrate the cells. Using a microscope, the number of reticulocytes per 1,000 red blod cells is determined.

Possible Interfering Materials and Conditions. None reported yet.

Normal Range. 0.1 to 1.5 reticulocytes per 100 red blood cells.

White Cell Count

White blood cells (leucocytes) are important in the defense of the body against invading microorganisms, since they destroy most harmful bacteria. An increase in the count is usually seen in infections. It may also be observed in other conditions including emotional upsets, blood disorders, and anesthesia. A decrease in the white blood cells may be seen in blood dyscrasias, overwhelming infections, and drug and chemical toxicity.

Food and Restrictions. None.

Procedure for Performing Test and Collecting Specimen. Essentially the same as for the red blood cell count, but a different pipette is used with a special diluting solution to hemolyze the red cells.

Possible Interfering Materials and Conditions. None reported yet.

Normal Range. 4000 to 11,000 per cubic mm.

White Cell Differential Count

There are several kinds of white blood cells (leucocytes) which can be identified microscopically. It is often helpful to know whether the proportions of these cells in the blood have changed, inasmuch as that may direct attention to a particular group of diseases. The neutrophiles (neutral staining multinucleated cells) are increased in most bacterial infections. The eosinophiles (acid staining multinucleated cells) are increased in parasitic infestations and allergic conditions. The basophiles (basic staining multinucleated cells) may be increased in some blood dyscrasias. The lymphocytes may be increased in measles and in several bacterial infections. The monocytes may be increased during recovery from severe infections, Hodgkin's disease, and lipoid storage diseases. The reasons for these changes are not known.

Food and Drink Restrictions. None.

Procedure for Performing Test and Collecting Specimen. A drop of fresh blood is placed on a slide and, using a second slide, is spread evenly over the surface of the glass in a thin film. After the film has dried, it is stained and examined under the microscope. Each type of white blood cell is counted separately. A total of 100 white cells of all kinds is counted, and the relative percentage of each calculated.

Possible Interfering Materials and Conditions. None reported yet.

Normal Range:

Neutrophiles	54% to 62%
Eosinophiles (acidophiles)	1% to 3%
Basophiles	0% to 1%
Lymphocytes	25% to 33%
Monocytes	0% to 9%

Blood Types

Blood typing tests are important in patients who may need blood transfusions and in pregnant women. There are four main blood types, A, B, AB, and O, and several minor types. The letters refer to the kind of agglutinogen present in the red blood cells. Type A blood has A agglutinogen, B has B agglutinogen. AB has both A and B agglutinogen, and O has no agglutinogen. Each person has in his *serum* the agglutinins which react with all types of *agglutinogen not present* in his own cells. Thus A blood has anti-B agglutinin, B blood has anti-A agglutinin, AB has *no* agglutinin, and O has both anti-A and anti-B agglutinins. Whenever agglutinins in sufficient concentration come in contact with the corresponding agglutinogen, agglutination (clumping) of the red cells occurs, followed by rapid destruction of these cells. This often causes death. Thus if A blood is mixed with B or O type in equal amounts, the anti-A agglutinins in the other blood will clump and destroy the A cells. In most cases of incompatible transfusion, it is the *donor's* cells which are agglutinated by the recipient's (patient's) serum, rather than the reverse. The reason for this is that in a transfusion 500 cc. of donor's blood are added to approximately 5000 cc. of recipient's blood. The donor's blood is, therefore, diluted approximately 10 times. This weakens the agglutinins of the donor's blood so that ordinarily they cannot agglutinate red cells.

However, the agglutinins of the recipient's blood are only diluted by 10 *per cent,* and remain strong. The dilution of the donor's blood does not affect the agglutinogens of the donor's red cells. Thus, the agglutinins of the recipient will clump the red cells of the donor in most incompatible transfusions. Exceptions occur only in those cases in which the donor has an unusually high concentration of agglutinins in his serum (higher titer). In these rare cases the donor's agglutinins are powerful enough to remain active even after a 1:10 dilution and will clump the recipient's red cells.

It is usually advisable to transfuse only with the same type of blood as that of the recipient. However, in emergencies, type O blood (universal donor) is sometimes given to patients with different blood types. In most cases this is safe because the O cells of the donor have no agglutinogens and cannot be clumped by the recipient's serum. Also the 1:10 dilution of the donor's serum usually prevents it from clumping the recipient's red cells. There is, however, always the danger that the donor's serum may have a high agglutinin titer and clump the patient's blood. Therefore, when type O blood is given to patients of a different blood type, it is done as a calculated risk. In these cases constant observation of the patient is essential thoroughout the *entire* transfusion so that it may be stopped at once if a reaction occurs.

In a similar fashion the AB blood is called "universal recipient" and can usually receive blood of any type. Here, too, if the titer of the agglutinins in the donor's blood is high, a severe or even fatal reaction may occur. The same considerations and precautions that apply to the use of "universal donor" blood also apply, therefore, to "universal recipients" receiving blood of different types.

In recent years additional blood types have been found and probably more will be discovered. These other types exist in conjunction with the main groups and the Rh groups. Their importance is much less, although they have theoretical interest and are sometimes used with the other groups in cases of disputed paternity.

Rh Factor

The Rh factor is found in conjunction with any one of the main blood types. A person may be ARh+, ARh−, BRh+, BRh−, etc. The presence of the Rh factor is designated Rh+, its absence Rh−. The same considerations which apply to the main groups also apply to the Rh groups in transfusions. The Rh groups differ from the main blood groups in two important respects. First, the serum of an Rh− person does not ordinarily have significant amounts of anti-Rh agglutinins, unless there has been previous exposure to Rh+ blood. The previous exposure may have been a transfusion or injection of Rh+ blood, or pregnancy with an Rh+ fetus. With exposure to Rh+ blood, the Rh− person gradually builds up a high titer of anti-Rh agglutinins. The second difference between the Rh and main blood groupings is that in some cases anti-Rh agglutinin readily crosses the placental barrier, while the main agglutinins apparently do not usually do so in significant quantities. The importance of these aspects of the Rh factor lies not only in the area of blood transfusions, but also in pregnancy. The occurrence of erythroblastosis fetalis (destruction of the infant's red cells) in Rh+ babies born to Rh− mothers is commonly known and greatly exaggerated. Because of the need for prior exposure to Rh+ blood before large amounts of anti-Rh agglutinins are produced, the first Rh+ child of an Rh− mother will almost always be normal unless the mother has had a transfusion or injection of Rh+ blood. Also, many Rh− women have several normal Rh+ children, since there is considerable variation in the titer of anti-Rh agglutinin produced by different individuals and also in the amounts of anti-Rh agglutinin which pass the placental barrier.

Over 90 per cent of all infants born with erythroblastosis come from Rh negative mothers who have produced anti-Rh antibodies. The remainder result from immunization of the mother to one of the major blood groups (A and B) or to one of the minor blood groups.

In some hospitals, women with Rh− blood are tested for

rising titer of anti-Rh antibodies. This is sometimes, but not always, helpful in predicting the occurrence of erythroblastosis in the infant.

The Rh antigen is now referred to as the D antigen by some authorities.

Food and Drink Restrictions. None.

Procedure for Collecting Specimen. Venous blood is withdrawn and 5 cc. placed in a test tube and allowed to clot.

Laboratory Procedure. There are several methods of typing blood, each with its own advantages and disadvantages. In general, all methods depend on the mixing of the patient's red cells with separate standard serum samples of groups A and B. As an additional check, the patient's serum is mixed with red cell suspensions of A and also of B types. The type of serum which agglutinates the patient's red cells and the type of red cell agglutinated by the patient's serum indicate the patient's blood type. A similar test is used to distinguish between Rh− and Rh+ blood. False positive as well as false negative reactions can occur, so that these tests are entrusted to a skilled and experienced person. A mistake in blood typing may be responsible for the death of the patient.

Possible Interfering Materials and Conditions. None reported yet.

Blood Urea Nitrogen (B.U.N.)

See Urea Nitrogen

Bromsulphalein Retention (B.S.P.)

This is a sensitive test for liver function. When Bromsulphalein is injected intravenously, about 80 per cent of it is removed by the liver and about 20 per cent by other organs. If the liver does not function properly, a larger amount than normal of the injected Bromsulphalein will remain in the blood. If marked jaundice is present, the test cannot be performed satisfactorily and is not needed.

Recently, evidence has been obtained that Bromsulphalein is an irritant to the veins, and that in about 15 per cent of cases, some venous induration will occur, apparently on the basis of local thrombophlebitis. Accordingly, there have been warnings against use of the test except for clearly defined reasons.

Bromsulphalein may be particularly hazardous in patients with asthma.

There have also been reports of serious and fatal sensitivity reactions to Bromsulphalein. *Therefore, it is recommended that on the injection tray there be an extra syringe and needle, and an ampul of epinephrine.*

Food and Drink Restrictions. The patient must fast for 12 hours before the test. Water is permitted.

Procedure for Collecting Specimen. The patient cannot receive any other dyes for 2 days before the test, and must be fasting for 12 hours.

The solution must *not* be refrigerated and should be at room temperature. The vial should be examined in good light for possible crystals before the contents are injected. The injection itself should be done slowly, taking a full 3 minutes. The patient is weighed just before the test and 5 mg. of Bromsulphalein dye per kg. of body weight is injected intravenously by the physician. It is essential that none of the dye be allowed to leak into the tissues, since it is highly irritant and causes sloughing. After exactly 45 minutes have passed, 5 cc. of venous blood is withdrawn from the opposite arm, placed in a test tube, and allowed to coagulate. The test is performed on the serum.

Laboratory Procedure. The amount of Bromsulphalein in the serum sample is determined colorimetrically. Marked jaundice will make the measurements unsatisfactory.

Possible Interfering Materials and Conditions. The B.S.P. may be artificially elevated if the patient has taken any of a large variety of drugs. Because of the number of drugs involved, they are listed mainly by official (generic) name, with only a few prominent brand names included:

Amidone
Anabolic steroids
(see table 16)
Androgens (see table 16)
Antifungal agents
Aspidium
Azo drugs (see table 17)
Barbiturates (see table 18)
Bunamiodyl
Chlorpropamide
Chlortetracycline
Choleretics
Clofibrate
Clomiphene
Contraceptives, oral
Demerol
Dyes for gallbladder studies
Estradiol
Estriol
Estrogens (see table 21)
Ethoxazene
Florantyrone

Fluoxymesterone
Heparin
Iopanoic acid
Isocarboxazid
MAO inhibitors
Meperidine
Metaxalone
Methandrostenolone
Methotrexate
Methyldopa
Methyltestosterone
Morphine
Norethandrolone
Norethindrone
Oxacillin
Pethidine
Phenazopyridine
Phenolphthalein
Probenecid
Tolbutamide
Triacetyloleandomycin

Normal Range. Less than 0.4 mg of Bromsulphalein per 100 cc. of serum. If expressed as % retention, the normal level is less than 5%.

B.S.P.

See Bromsulphalein Retention

B.T.

See Bleeding Time

B.U.N.

See Urea Nitrogen

Calcium

Calcium is one of the essential ions in the body. It is needed for many vital processes such as muscular contraction, nerve transmission, and blood clotting. The minimum concentration of calcium ions required for each of these processes differs somewhat. Only ionized calcium is effective, and unfortunately there is no satisfactory method of measuring ionized calcium levels. However, the total amount of calcium, ionized and nonionized can be determined. It is generally believed that about 50 per cent of the total calcium is ionized. If there is any acidosis, the percentage of ionized calcium is higher. In alkalosis, the percentage of ionized calcium is lower. The total calcium level alone does not indicate the amount of ionized calcium.

When there is a deficiency in ionized calcium, the major manifestation is a generalized tetanic condition beginning with twitching of muscle fibers and finally producing tetanic convulsions. This condition is probably due to the response of the nerves or neuromuscular junctions to the reduced calcium levels. It is unlikely that blood clotting changes are related to calcium levels, since normal clotting can take place at calcium levels considerably lower than those which would be fatal because of the production of severe, sustained tetanic convulsions. Therefore, calcium determinations are of no value in disorders of blood clotting.

A decrease in the blood calcium, called hypocalcemia, occurs in several conditions. In celiac disease and sprue, absorption of calcium from the gastrointestinal tract is impaired. In hypoparathyroidism, the balance between blood calcium and bone calcium is disturbed, and in some kidney diseases excess calcium is lost in the urine.

An increase in the blood calcium (hypercalcemia) is found in a number of conditions, including hyperparathyroidism (overfunctioning of the parathyroids), multiple myeloma, and respiratory diseases with increased carbon dioxide tension (concentration) in the blood.

Food and Drink Restrictions. None.

Procedure for Collecting Specimen. Venous blood is withdrawn after the tourniquet has been released, and 6 cc. placed in a test tube and allowed to coagulate. Cork stoppers should not be used. The test is performed on the serum.

Laboratory Procedure. Two methods are generally in use. The chemical method involves the precipitation of calcium as the oxalate, followed by titration with potassium permanganate. Calcium levels may also be determined by flame photometry where suitable apparatus is available.

Possible Interfering Materials and Conditions. The serum calcium level may be spuriously decreased if the patient has had a BSP retention test during the previous 24 to 48 hours.

A number of drugs may interfere with the calcium measurement, making it difficult or impossible to obtain a correct reading. They include:

Heparin
Insulin
Magnesium salts

Normal Range:
9.0 to 11.5 mg. per 100 cc. of serum, or
4.5 to 5.8 milliequivalents per liter.

Carbon Dioxide CO_2

Carbon dioxide levels in plasma are measured in cases of suspected respiratory insufficiency. A higher than normal concentration of carbon dioxide may indicate that gas exchange is inadequate. This test is often performed, and interpreted in conjunction with the oxygen level (P.78) and pH (P.63) of the plasma.

Carbon dioxide levels are ordinarily measured in *venous* plasma. Under some circumstances, arterial carbon dioxide levels may be measured. The arterial levels are normally slightly different from venous levels, and the technique of obtaining arterial blood is more difficult, usually requiring a specially trained physician.

The physician may designate carbon dioxide level measurement "emergency."

Food and Drink Restrictions. None.

Procedure for Collecting Specimen. A heparinized vacutainer tube should be used, and *completely filled with blood.* If air gets into the tube, the results will be distorted. Sometimes it is possible to collect blood in a heparinized syringe, preferably plastic. The blood is then stored in a tube under mineral oil, although this may not be completely satisfactory. The amount of blood collected should be at least 4 cc., but more may be needed to fill the vacutainer tube completely. It is also vital that there be no fist-clenching or exercise of the arm that might raise carbon dioxide content.

Laboratory Procedure. The sample is acidified, and the carbon dioxide gas extracted and measured in a gasometer.

Possible Interfering Materials and Conditions. The test for carbon dioxide content may be interfered with if the patient has received:

> Dimercaprol
> Lipomul
> Methicillin

There may be a spurious decrease in carbon dioxide content if the patient has received nitrofurantoin.

Inadvertent exposure of the sample to outside air may give erroneus results. Exercise of the hand and forearm muscles may produce spurious elevations.

Normal Range. The normal range for *venous* plasma carbon dioxide as given by several authorities varies somewhat. Some give fairly narrow limits, others wider ones. The following range encompasses most of the figures given:

> 22 to 34 mM. per L. *or*
> 22 to 34 mEq. per L. *or*
> 50 to 60 vol. per cent.

The normal range for *arterial* plasma carbon dioxide is: 21 to 30 mM./L. or mEq./L.

Carbon Dioxide Combining Power

See CO_2 Combining Power

Carbon Monoxide

In suspected carbon monoxide poisoning, the identification of significant amounts of carbon monoxide in the blood establishes the diagnosis. The test is not restricted to acute carbon monoxide poisoning which frequently has a fatal outcome before the doctor arrives. There are many cases of chronic, low grade carbon monoxide poisoning causing such symptoms as headache, malaise and weakness. They are not easily diagnosed except by determination of the blood carbon monoxide level and usually result from occupational exposure to exhaust gases in industrial plants, garages, etc. They may also come from defective gas-burning appliances in the home. Most persons have small amounts of carbon monoxide in their blood from exposure to tobacco smoke, automobile exhaust fumes, etc.

There have been tragic deaths because this test was omitted on persons who came to hospital clinics in the winter complaining of headache. In at least one case, the patient went home, and the defective gas heater whose carbon monoxide output caused the headache killed all but one of the family that night.

Food and Drink Restrictions. None.

Procedure for Collecting Specimen. Venous blood is withdrawn and 5 cc. placed in an oxalate bottle or tube.

Laboratory Procedure. There are several laboratory procedures available. A usual method is quantitative estimation using a reversion spectroscope.

Possible Interfering Materials and Conditions. None reported yet.

Normal Range. Less than 0.8 volume per cent of blood.

CBC

See Blood Counts

Cephalin Flocculation

This test is useful in diagnosing liver damage. The serum of normal persons, properly diluted, will not flocculate (clump) a colloidal suspension of cephalin and cholesterol. On the other hand, the serum of persons whose liver cells are damaged does flocculate the suspension. This test is sensitive and frequently positive in the early stages of liver disease before jaundice appears. It is negative in acute obstruction of the biliary tract of short duration. If the obstruction persists, secondary damage to the liver cells occurs and the cephalin flocculation test becomes positive. Certain types of liver disease which do not damage the liver cells give a negative reaction, for example, neoplasms and abscesses. Some nonhepatic disorders, such as malaria, kala-azar, and rheumatoid arthritis, may sometimes produce a positive reaction. A positive test, therefore, is not itself conclusive. Since this test affords a rough quantitative measurement of liver cell function, it is sometimes used to follow the course of patients with a known liver disease, such as cirrhosis. The results are reported as negative to 4+.

Food and Drink Restrictions. None.

Procedure for Collecting Specimen. Venous blood is withdrawn and 5 cc. placed in a test tube and allowed to coagulate. The test is performed on the serum.

Laboratory Procedure. A 1:20 dilution of the serum is added to a suspension of cephalin and cholesterol. The extent of flocculation is observed at the end of 24 and 48 hours.

Possible Interfering Materials and Conditions. Both false positive and false negative reactions may occur if the patient is taking methyldopa (Aldomet, Aldoril).

Normal Range. Either negative or 1+. Reports are delayed 24 to 48 hours.

Chlorides

Chlorides are measured to help diagnose disorders in the maintenance of normal osmotic relationships, acid-base balance, and water balance of the body. Usually this test is performed together with measurement of other ions of the blood.

An elevation in blood chlorides (hyperchloremia) occurs in several conditions, including various kidney disorders, Cushing's syndrome, and hyperventilation. A decrease in blood chlorides (hypochloremia) is seen in such states as excessive vomiting and diarrhea, diabetic acidosis, Addison's disease, heat exhaustion, and following certain surgical procedures.

Food and Drink Restrictions. None.

Procedure for Collecting Specimen. Venous blood is withdrawn and 5 cc. placed in a test tube and allowed to clot. The test is performed on the serum.

Laboratory Procedure. The chlorides are precipitated by silver iodate, leaving a soluble iodate which is titrated with sodium thiosulfate.

Possible Interfering Materials and Conditions. There may be an apparent elevation of chloride if the patient has been taking bromides (Fello-Sed, Neurosine).

Normal Range. This may be expressed in various ways:
100 to 106 milliequivalents per liter of serum, or
355 to 376 mg. of chloride per 100 cc. of serum, or
585 to 620 mg. of *sodium chloride* per 100 cc. of serum or plasma.

Cholesterol

Cholesterol is a normal constituent of the blood and is found in all cells but its exact physiologic function is not clear. It may serve as the substance from which various hormones are synthesized. In various disease states the cholesterol concentration in the serum may be raised or lowered. Cholesterol levels are elevated in many conditions; in most the finding is only incidental. An elevated cholesterol level may be helpful in the diagnosis of xanthomatosis, certain liver diseases, and hypothyroidism. There is also increasing interest in the role of cholesterol in producing myocardial infarction since deposits of cholesterol, known as plaques, are often found partially blocking the coronary arteries. However, there is as yet no conclusive evidence linking this condition to the blood serum cholesterol concentration. Decreased serum cholesterol is found in hyperthyroidism, anemias, starvation, and acute infections.

Food and Drink Restrictions. Serum cholesterol levels are not influenced by diet over a short period of time, although they are affected over a long period of time. Therefore, fasting is *not* required before taking the sample. However, it would probably be prudent to avoid foods containing large amounts of cholesterol for the 12 hours preceding the test. Such foods are egg yolk and brains.

Procedure for Collecting Specimen. Venous blood is withdrawn and 5 cc. placed in a test tube and allowed to coagulate. The test is performed on the serum.

Laboratory Procedure. Total cholesterol is hydrolyzed with alkali and precipitated with digitonin. The precipitate is redissolved and reagents added which produce a color. The color intensity, measured with a colorimeter, is proportional to the concentration. This test usually takes about 48 hours.

Possible Interfering Materials and Conditions. The cholesterol level may be spuriously elevated if the patient has taken any of the following:

Bile salts	Metandienone
Bromides	Vitamin A

Another drug, diphenylhydantoin (Dilantin), may also elevate cholesterol levels, but it is not known whether this is an interference or a pharmacologic effect.

Certain antibiotics, notably the tetracyclines and neomycin, may produce a true, but temporary and misleading reduction in cholesterol levels.

Anoxia may increase serum cholesterol levels.

Normal Range. 120 to 260 mg. per 100 cc. of serum.

Many persons over the age of 30 have cholesterol levels that are higher than 260 mg./100 cc. It has been suggested that the upper limit of normal be considered about 360 mg./100 cc. We do not know whether the higher levels in people over 30 are truly normal, physiological and harmless, or whether substantial numbers of these people already have atherosclerosis, and that this is reflected in the cholesterol level. It will take years to resolve this problem in interpretation.

Cholesterol Esters

In addition to free cholesterol, there are cholesterol esters in the serum. Their physiologic role is unknown. The proportion of cholesterol esters is normal in some xanthomatoses. The proportion of esters is low in some obstructions of the common bile duct, but the total amount is normal. In cases where liver cells are damaged, there is a drop in both absolute and relative amounts of the esters. The determination of the esters may therefore be helpful in assessing the amount of cellular damage in the liver.

Food and Drink Restrictions. See cholesterol.

Procedure for Collecting Specimen. Venous blood is withdrawn and 7 cc. placed in a test tube and allowed to coagulate. The test is performed on the serum.

Laboratory Procedure. Total cholesterol is measured as described above. On another sample, the free cholesterol is determined by following the same procedure but omitting hydrolysis with alkali. The difference between free and total cholesterol values represents the quantity of cholesterol esters. This test usually requires about one week.

Possible Interfering Materials and Conditions. None reported yet.

Normal Range. 60 to 80 percent of the total cholesterol.

Clotting (Coagulation) Time

This test measures the ability of blood to clot. Many factors are involved in clotting, including prothrombin, thromboplastin, and fibrinogen. New clotting factors are continually being discovered. A deficiency of any essential factor or an increase in inhibitory factors may prolong clotting time. This test is distinct from the bleeding time test since the latter also involves the ability of small blood vessels to constrict. This test, furthermore, should not be confused with special clotting time measurements that use siliconized or lusteroid test tubes.

Food and Drink Restrictions. None.

Procedure for Performing Test and Collecting Specimen. There are several methods. The most common ones involve the use of venous blood. Freshly drawn blood is put into 4 small test tubes (1 cc. in each) and the first tube is tilted at 30-second intervals. When clotting is observed, the same procedure is followed in succession with the other 3 tubes. The clotting time is the average of the times elapsed between venipuncture and clotting in the last 3 tubes.

Possible Interfering Materials and Conditions. None reported yet.

Normal Range. 10 to 25 minutes *by this method.* Using other methods of measurement, normal clotting time may be 1 to 5 minutes.

Coagulation

See Clotting Time

CO_2 Combining Power

This test is a general measure of the acidity or alkalinity of the blood. An increase in CO_2 combining power is usually a manifestation of alkalosis, while a decrease is usually a manifestation of acidosis. However, changes in CO_2 combining power do not always represent changes in pH of the blood, since the latter depends on the ratio, not on the absolute amounts, of basic and acidic substances. As in many other tests, good clinical judgment is needed to evaluate the results. High CO_2 combining power is usually found in conditions such as persistent vomiting or drainage of the stomach with loss of hydrochloric acid, excessive intake of sodium bicarbonate in the presence of poor kidney function, excessive administration of ACTH or cortisone, and hypoventilation. Low CO_2 combining power is usually found in such conditions as diabetic acidosis, severe diarrhea or drainage of intestinal fluids, certain kidney diseases, and hyperventilation. In many cases it is also necessary to test the pH of the blood to evaluate properly the acid-base balance. The CO_2 combining power test may, in some situations, be designated by the physician as "emergency."

Food and Drink Restrictions. None.

Procedure for Collecting Specimen. Venous blood should be withdrawn without using a tourniquet, if possible. If a tourniquet is necessary, the patient should *not* open and close his fist, but should keep it closed without straining. For years, the blood sample was collected under oil. However, there is a growing trend away from oil. Instead, vacuum tubes containing heparin are used, and 7 cc. of blood collected in them. In some hospitals, oiled syringes are still used, and can give satisfactory results.

Laboratory Procedure. Usually the Van Slyke apparatus is used. The serum sample is equilibrated with alveolar air. Then the carbon dioxide, combined with the serum, is freed by adding an acid and the volume measured.

Possible Interfering Materials and Conditions. The carbon dioxide combining power may be spuriously decreased if the patient has taken nitrofurantoin.

Normal Range:
53 to 78 volumes per 100 cc. of serum, or
24 to 35 milliequivalents per liter of serum.

Congo Red Retention

This is a test for amyloidosis. In this disease deposits of amyloid tissue are laid down in such organs as liver, kidneys and spleen, and eventually interfere with proper function. The amyloid material has an affinity for Congo red and removes it from the blood. In patients with amyloid disease, therefore, the dye disappears from the blood more rapidly than in normal humans. In advanced amyloidosis 60 to 99 per cent of the dye may be removed in 4 minutes. The test may be negative in the early stages of the disease. In fact, up to 50 per cent of patients with amyloidosis may have negative Congo red tests.

Food and Drink Restrictions. None.

Procedure for Performing Test and Collecting Specimen. At least 2 days must elapse between the injection of any other dye, such as BSP, and this test. The physician injects intravenously 0.3 cc. of a 1% solution of Congo red per kg. of body weight, completing the injection within 1 minute. Exactly 5 minutes later, 6 cc. of venous blood is drawn from the opposite arm and placed in a test tube, where it coagulates. Exactly 1 hour after the injection of the dye another 6 cc. sample of venous blood is drawn and placed in another test tube. After the second blood sample has been collected, a specimen of urine is also obtained.

Laboratory Procedure. The amount of dye in the serum is determined colorimetrically.

Possible Interfering Materials and Conditions. If the patient has albuminuria associated with hypoproteinemia there may be a false positive reaction.

Normal Range. Less than 40 per cent of the injected dye disappears from the blood in 1 hour.

Coombs' Direct

This is also called a direct antiglobulin test. It is a basic immunologic procedure which reveals antigen-antibody reactions that are, in a sense, incomplete or weak. For example, antibodies to human red cells may combine with the red cells in such a way as to damage them, or increase their fragility but not cause visible agglutination. Such antibodies are demonstrated by Coombs' test. It may be used in a wide variety of clinical or microbiological applications. Its major clinical uses, however, are in the early diagnosis of erythroblastosis fetalis (see P. 203), and autoimmune hemolytic anemia. A positive direct Coombs' test indicates that some antibody is attached to the red cells, but does not indicate the exact nature of the antibody. Many different diseases may produce a positive direct Coombs'.

Food and Drink Restrictions. None.

Procedure for Collecting Specimen. Fresh clotted blood is considered superior by several authorities. Venous blood may be used or, in the case of newborns, blood from the umbilical cord. Usually 2 cc. of blood is sufficient.

Laboratory Procedure. A washed suspension of the patient's red blood cells is added to some Coombs' serum (rabbit anti-human globulin) purchased from a reliable biological supply house. The red cells are then observed for agglutination. Results may be reported as 1 + to 4 +.

Possible Interfering Materials and Conditions. Many drugs can produce a positive direct Coombs' test. It is not clear whether this is an interference of a pharmacologic effect. The drugs, listed by official (generic) name include:

Aminopyrine
Cephaloridine
Cephalothin (effect may persist for months)
Methyldopa (effect may persist for months)
Penicillin (effect may persist for months)

Heparin may interfere in cases of acquired hemolytic anemia, and produce a negative direct Coombs'.

Normal Range. Normally, the direct Coombs' test is negative.

Coombs' Indirect

The indirect Coombs' test is used in detection of the various minor blood type factors, including Rh. If red cells of known antigenic composition (i.e., the minor blood type factors) are used, the related antibody content of a test serum can be determined. The reverse procedure may also be used. In cross-matching blood for transfusions, this test may be used to eliminate bloods which might cause reactions because of incompatibilities of the minor blood type factors.

Food and Drink Restrictions. None.

Procedure for Collecting Specimen. Fresh clotted blood is considered superior by several authorities. Usually 5 cc. of blood is sufficient.

Laboratory Procedure. Donor red cells and recipient serum are mixed together and allowed to stand. Then the red cells are removed and washed and antiglobulin is added. The reaction may be reported from 1+ to 4+.

Possible Interfering Materials and Conditions. None reported yet.

Normal Range. Usually the test is negative.

CPK

See Creatine Phosphokinase

C-Reactive Protein (C.R.P.)

The C-reactive protein test is a test for inflammation and tissue breakdown. Thus it is nonspecific and similar to the sedimentation rate test (*see* P.110). The C-reactive protein test is positive in myocardial infarction, acute rheumatic fever, widespread cancer, malaria, bacterial infection, and other conditions. It is sometimes used to follow the activity of a disease. The term C-reactive protein was chosen because the protein involved forms a precipitate with the C-polysaccharide of the pneumococcus. The relationship between this action and its use in diagnosis is not clear, and the clinical use of the test is based on the empirical observation that it is positive in conditions with widespread inflammation and tissue breakdown.

Food and Drink Restrictions. None.

Procedure for Collecting Specimen. There are two separate procedures in use. If the test is to be performed in the laboratory, clotted blood is needed. Venous blood is withdrawn and 5 cc. placed in a test tube and allowed to coagulate. The test is performed on the serum.

If the test is to be performed at the bedside, a fingertip

technique may be used. Special capillary tubes are used, and capillary blood is drawn into the tube and allowed to clot. After standing, the clot is discarded, leaving the serum for the test.

Laboratory Procedure. A sample of the serum is mixed with C-reactive protein antiserum. If a precipitate forms, the test is positive.

Possible Interfering Materials and Conditions. None reported yet.

Normal Range. No C-reactive protein present.

Creatine Phosphokinase (CPK)

This test is useful in the diagnosis of two quite different diseases, myocardial infarction and muscular dystrophy. The enzyme is found in both cardiac and skeletal muscle. In myocardial infarction, the rise in serum creatine phosphokinase may start in about four hours, and in 24 to 36 hours reach a peak at which the levels may be 50 to 100 times the normal levels. In early muscular dystrophy, often before clinical signs are clear, the creatine phosphokinase levels may be 300 to 400 times normal.

Food and Drink Restrictions. None reported yet.

Procedure for Collecting Specimen. Venous blood is withdrawn and 4 cc. placed in a test tube and allowed to coagulate. The test is performed on the serum. At times, the physician may designate this test "emergency."

Laboratory Procedure. Several different methods of measuring creatine phosphokinase levels are available.

Possible Interfering Materials and Conditions. Severe exercise may produce moderate increases in creatine phosphokinase levels, but not usually enough to mimic the serious diseases for which the test is used. Any condition causing severe muscle destruction, such as crush syndrome, may result in high levels. Slight elevations occur in dermatomyositis, delirum tremens, and hypothyroidism.

For reasons that are still unclear, some cases of pulmonary

infarction and pulmonary edema may have high creatine phosphokinase levels.

Electrocautery used within the preceding few days may also produce elevated levels.

Slight muscle injury, such as that produced by intramuscular injections, can also elevate the creatine phosphokinase.

Normal Range. This may be expressed in several ways, depending on the method of assay used and the institution. Thus one must know the range considered normal by the laboratory doing the measurement. Examples of normal ranges are:

> 5 to 44 units
> 0 to 5 microgm./hr./ml.
> Under 35 units
> 0 to 4 units

Creatinine

This test is a measurement of kidney function similar to the urea nitrogen test. Creatinine is derived from the breakdown of muscle creatine phosphate. The amount produced per day is relatively constant, and it is excreted by the kidney. An elevated blood creatinine level indicates a disorder of kidney function.

Food and Drink Restrictions. None.

Procedure for Collecting Specimen. Venous blood is withdrawn and 6 cc. placed in a test tube and allowed to coagulate. The test is performed on the serum.

Laboratory Procedure. To the serum sample is added alkaline picrate. The color produced is compared to standards and the concentration of creatinine calculated.

Possible Interfering Materials and Conditions. A spuriously high level of serum creatinine may result if the patient has had either a B.S.P. (Bromsulphalein) or P.S.P. (phenolsulfonphthalein) test within the previous 24 hours.

In addition, several drugs can produce spuriously high

levels. The drugs, listed by generic name, include:

Ascorbic acid
Barbiturates   Chlordiazepoxide

Spuriously low levels may be produced by methyldopa.
Normal Range. 0.6 to 1.3 per 100 cc. of serum.

C.T.

See Clotting Time

Culture

See Blood Culture, Chapter 2

Differential Count

See Blood Counts, White Cell Differential Count

Erythrocyte Count

See Blood Counts, Red Cell Count

E.S.R.

See Sedimentation Rate

Fasting Blood Sugar (F.B.S.)

See Glucose (Sugar)

Fibrinogen

In conditions characterized by inadequate blood clotting
it may be helpful to determine which element of the clotting
mechanism is deficient. The fibrinogen of the plasma is essential for blood clotting. In the presence of thrombin it is
converted to insoluble fibrin threads. Measurement of the
blood fibrinogen level may aid in establishing the cause of a
clotting deficiency.

Food and Drink Restrictions. None.

Procedure for Collecting Specimen. Venous blood is withdrawn and 5 cc. placed in an oxalate tube or bottle. Other

acceptable anticoagulants are EDTA and heparin. The test is performed on the plasma.

Laboratory Procedure. To the sample of plasma is added sodium sulfite which precipitates the fibrinogen. The amount of fibrinogen is measured by the biuret test.

Possible Interfering Materials and Conditions. None reported yet.

Normal Range. 200 to 600 mg. per 100 cc. of plasma. Plasma normally contains more fibrinogen than is actually needed for satisfactory clotting. Deficiencies in blood clotting due to fibrinogen deficiency do not occur until the concentration falls to 75 mg. per 100 cc. of plasma.

FTA-ABS

See Fluorescent Treponemal Antibody Absorption

Gammopathies

See Plasma Electrophoresis for Gammopathies

Globulin

See Albumin, Globulin, Total Protein, A/G Ratio

Glucose (Sugar)

This test is performed to discover whether there is a disorder of glucose metabolism. An increase in blood glucose level is found in severe diabetes, chronic liver disease, and overactivity of several of the endocrine glands. A symptom caused directly by the elevated blood sugar is occasional, intermittent blurring of vision. In mild diabetes there may be a normal glucose level, so that more sensitive tests need to be performed (*see Glucose Tolerance*). There may be a decrease in blood sugar in tumors of the islets of Langerhans in the pancreas, underfunctioning of various endocrine glands, glycogen storage disease (von Gierke's), and overtreatment with insulin. If the blood glucose level falls too low, coma, convulsions, and even death may result.

Food and Drink Restrictions. The patient must fast for 12 hours before the test. Water is permitted.

Procedure for Collecting Specimen. Venous blood is withdrawn and 3 to 5 cc. placed in an oxalate tube or bottle. Other acceptable anticoagulants are heparin, sodium fluoride and EDTA.

Laboratory Procedure. After precipitation of proteins the glucose in the filtrate is oxidized with cupric or ferricyanide solution. The amount present is then determined colorimetrically.

Possible Interfering Materials and Conditions. The blood glucose levels may be high if the patient has taken ACTH, physostigmine, or an overdose of nalidixic acid (Neg Gram).

If the o-toluidine method is used to measure glucose, the administration of dextrans to the patient may give spuriously high levels.

Normal Range. 80 to 120 mg. per 100 cc. of serum or 70 to 105 mg. per 100 cc. of whole blood.

G6PD

See Glucose-6-phosphate Dehydrogenase Test

Glucose-6-phosphate Dehydrogenase Test (G6PD)

This is test for congenital deficiency of the enzyme, glucose-6-phosphate dehydrogenase in the red blood cells. Acute hemolytic anemia may develop in patients with such a deficiency when certain drugs (such as primaquine) or foods (such as fava beans) are taken. A knowledge of the existence of this congenital deficiency can be helpful in advising the patient about avoidance of substances that can precipitate hemolytic anemia, and also for genetic counseling.

Food and Drink Restrictions. None.

Procedure for Collecting Specimen. Several are available. One requires the collection of a small amount of capillary blood in a heparinized microhematocrit tube. Another requires the collection of 4 cc. of venous blood which is placed in a test tube containing an anticoagulant. The laboratory of each institution should be asked which procedure it requires.

Laboratory Procedure. Several different laboratory procedures are available.

Possible Interfering Materials and Conditions. None reported yet.

Normal Range. Normally, the tests show substantial amounts (by color or staining techniques) of glucose-6-phosphate dehydrogenase in the red cells.

Glucose Tolerance

These tests are used to discover disorders of glucose metabolism which have not become severe enough to change the blood glucose levels in the fasting state. In the glucose tolerance tests, a large amount of glucose is given to a fasting patient, either intravenously or orally. At regular intervals thereafter, the blood glucose levels are measured to learn how long it takes the body to handle the added glucose. If it remains in the blood for an excessive period of time, there is some disorder of carbohydrate metabolism. The intravenous test is somewhat more sensitive than the oral, since the factor of absorption from the gastrointestinal tract is not involved. In the oral test, an increase in blood sugar and its persistence for 3 hours is seen in diabetes. In the intravenous test the blood sugar is, of course, elevated in all cases. If the blood glucose concentration does not return to normal within less than 3 hours after the intravenous administration of glucose, diabetes is probably present. If 1 to 2 hours are required to return to normal there may be some liver disorder. The urine voided during the course of this test is examined for sugar to obtain additional information about the kidney excretion of excess sugar.

Food and Drink Restrictions. The patient should be on an adequate diet, containing at least 150 gm. of carbohydrate per day for at least one week. For 12 hours before the test, the patient must fast, but may have water ad lib.

Procedure for Collecting Specimen. The following steps are taken in order:

1. Withdraw venous blood and place 3 cc. in an oxalate or fluoride bottle or tube supplied by the laboratory.
2. Collect urine specimen at once.
3. If the intravenous test is used the doctor will administer intravenously by slow infusion 0.5 Gm. of glucose per kg. of body weight. He will use a 20% solution and take 30 minutes for the infusion.
3a. If the oral test is used, the patient receives 1.75 Gm. of glucose per kg. of body weight in unsweetened lemonade. There are also available commercial preparations containing the appropriate amounts of glucose in beverages or gels.
4. If the intravenous test is used, 3 cc. of venous blood is withdrawn immediately from the arm which did not receive the infusion; subsequent withdrawals are made exactly 30, 60, 90 and 150 minutes following the infusion. The blood is placed in an oxalate or fluoride bottle or tube. With each sample, a urine specimen is collected.
4a. In the oral test, 3 cc. of venous blood is collected 30, 60, 120 and 180 minutes after ingestion of the glucose and placed in an oxalate bottle or tube. With each blood sample a urine specimen is also collected.
5. Each specimen must be labeled with the date and time of collection.

Laboratory Procedure. The laboratory will test each blood sample as described under *Glucose* and each urine sample as described under *Sugar, Qualitative, Chapter 5.*

Possible Interfering Materials and Conditions. The glucose tolerance curve may be altered if the patient has taken any of the following:

> Isocarboxazid
> Oral contraceptives
> Phenelzine

Normal Range:
Oral: Peak of not more than 150 mg. per 100 cc. of serum; return to fasting within 2 hours.
Intravenous: Return to fasting level within about 1 hour.

Recent evidence suggests that the above criteria may be much too strict for middle-aged and elderly subjects. In a reappraisal, West considers that for patients over 59 years of age, one hour values as high as 200 mg. % may be within normal limits.

Grouping

See Blood Types

GT

See Glucose Tolerance

GTT

See Glucose Tolerance Test

Guthrie

This is a blood test for the presence of phenylketonuria. It is used as a general screening procedure for young infants before they leave the hospital. It is useful on infants as young as two days, and is generally performed between the second and third days of life, although it can be performed on older infants also. The Guthrie test has one advantage over the urine test for phenylketonuria (see page 124). The urine test is not ordinarily significant until the age of three weeks, and by that time, the infant has usually left the hospital.

A negative Guthrie test means that there is no appreciable danger of phenylketonuria. A positive test does not definitely establish phenylketonuria, but means that there is a considerable chance of its being present. If the Guthrie test is positive, a more intricate test-measurement of blood phenylalanine levels is ordinarily necessary; however this is not usually done in the average hospital but in specially equipped laboratories.

The Guthrie test is one of the tests which is legally acceptable for phenylketonuria in those states which require testing of all newborns for the disease.

Food and Drink Restrictions. None.

Procedure for Collecting Specimen. The heel of the infant is pricked with a disposable lancet and three drops of blood are collected on a piece of special filter paper furnished by the laboratory.

The blood specimen must be collected no earlier than the third day of life, and no earlier than 48 hours after the start of feeding with milk or protein-containing substitute.

Laboratory Procedure. The filter paper is autoclaved, and a small circle punched from the center of a blood-stain. This small punch-out is then placed on the surface of a Petri dish containing nutrient agar mixed with a substrate that inhibits Bacillus subtilis, and well streaked with a culture of that bacillus. If the bacillus does not grow near the blood-stained filter paper, the test is negative. If the bacillus does grow near the filter paper, the test is positive.

Possible Interfering Materials and Conditions. None reported yet.

Normal Range. Normally, the Guthrie test is negative.

Hb

See Hemoglobin

Hgb

See Hemoglobin

Heat Stable Lactic Dehydrogenase (HLDH)

This test is used primarily as an aid in the diagnosis of myocardial infarction in cases in which the regular lactic dehydrogenase test may not be sufficiently specific. Latic dehydrogenase, of which at least 5 different types are known, is found in serum and in several organs. Thus an elevated level of latic dehydrogenase might result from a variety of conditions (P.85). It has been found that one type of lactic dehydrogenase is stable when heated in a particular manner and that it is more specific in cases of myocardial infarction than are the others. Consequently, when the diagnosis is in doubt, a heat stable lactic dehydrogenase test may be done.

Food and Drink Restrictions. None reported.

Procedure for Collecting Specimen. Venous blood is withdrawn and 6 ml. placed in a test tube and allowed to coagulate. Hemolysis must be avoided.

Laboratory Procedure. A specimen of the serum is kept at a fixed, elevated temperature for a fixed period of time. Then the enzyme activity is measured as described under lactic dehydrogenase.

Possible Interfering Materials and Conditions. If any oxalate comes in contact with the specimen, it will cause falsely low readings. Megaloblastic anemia, hemolytic anemia, and muscular dystrophy may produce false positive results.

Normal Range. The normal range is not precisely known. In general, experts consider values below 115 units not clearly diagnostic of myocardial infarction, while values over 115 units generally are.

Hematocrit

This test measures the relative volume of cells and plasma in the blood. In anemias and after hemorrhage the hematocrit reading is lowered; in polycythemia and dehydration it is raised.

Food and Drink Restrictions. None.

Procedure for Collecting Specimen. Venous blood is withdrawn and 4 cc. placed in an oxalate tube or bottle. Other acceptable anticoagulants are heparin and EDTA.

Laboratory Procedure. The oxalated blood is carefully placed in a special (Wintrobe) tube up to the 0 mark. The tube is then spun in a centrifuge and the height of the col-

umn of packed red blood cells measured against the grada-
tions on the side of the tube.

Possible Interfering Materials and Conditions. None reported yet.

Normal Range:

Men, 40 to 50 mm. of red blood cells per 100 mm. of column
    height;

Women, 35 to 45 mm.

Hemoglobin

Hemoglobin, the essential oxygen carrier of the blood, is
found within the red blood cells and is responsible for the
red color of the blood. The hemoglobin is decreased in hemorrhage and anemias and increased in hemoconcentration
and polycythemia. The hemoglobin and red cell count do
not always rise or fall equally. This fact is often important
in differential diagnosis of anemias. In iron deficiency (microcytic) anemia, hemoglobin is reduced more than the red
blood cell count. In pernicious anemia, the red cell count is
reduced more than hemoglobin.

Food and Drink Restrictions. None.

Procedure for Performing Test and Collecting Specimen.
Capillary blood is employed.

The older procedure is the Sahli method. The finger or
ear lobe is punctured and blood drawn into a special pipette
up to a mark. The blood is then placed in a special graduated
test tube and diluted hydrochloric acid added, converting
the hemoglobin to acid hematin. The mixture is then diluted until it matches the color of a standard. The amount
of hemoglobin is determined by measuring the height of the
fluid column against the graduations on the side of the test
tube. Many laboratories now use photometric techniques to
measure hemoglobin.

Possible Interfering Materials and Conditions. None reported yet.

Normal Range. 12 to 18 Gm. per 100 cc. of blood.

Hemoglobin Electrophoresis

This is a test to identify abnormal hemoglobins. There are at least 150 different hemoglobins, most of them differing from the common hemoglobin only by a single amino acid. These abnormal hemoglobins are genetically transmitted and a patient may have two of them, one from each parent. Not all of them produce clinical symptoms. The most common one (Hb S), produces sickling (P.115). The most common clinical sign of the presence of abnormal hemoglobins is anemia that is resistant to ordinary treatment. The hemoglobins are designated by a series of letters, numbers, and subscripts that are related to their mobility during electrophoresis and to where they were discovered. Normal hemoglobin is hemoglobin A (Hb A). Abnormal hemoglobins are Hb D, Hb E, Hb A$_2$ Hb M$_{Boston}$ and so forth.

Food and Drink Restrictions. None.

Procedure for Collecting Specimen. The patient should not have had a blood transfusion during the preceding four months. Venous blood is withdrawn and 4 ml. put into a tube containing an anticoagulant.

Laboratory Procedure. The red cells are washed and then hemolysed. The hemolysed material is subjected to electrophoresis and the bands compared to known standards.

Possible Interfering Materials and Conditions. A blood transfusion given during the preceding four months may cause the results to be spurious.

Normal Range. Normally, only hemoglobin A is present in adults. In infants, hemoglobin F is also present.

Hepatitis Test

This is a test of bank blood for the presence of the Australia antigen which generally indicates the presence of the serum hepatitis virus. Since serum hepatitis is the most serious complication of blood transfusions, with a mortality rate of 5 to 10 %, it is vital to be able to detect blood that can cause this disease. In volunteer blood donors, between 1 and 2 in every 1,000 are positive; in commercial blood donors, 10 to 12 in every 1,000 are positive. Since millions of blood transfusions are given each year, the savings in lives and disability from eliminating the contaminated blood from banks is substantial. Every blood bank should employ this test routinely on each and every unit of blood. False positives are virtually unknown, and false negatives are rare. The test is generally performed on bank blood that has already been drawn from the donor.

Food and Drink Restrictions. None.

Procedure for Collecting Specimen. A sample of the bank blood is used.

Laboratory Procedure. The serum sample is subjected to high voltage immunoelectroosmophoresis (IEOP), with serum from persons known to have high antibody titers to the hepatitis (Australia) antigen. Tests are run on many samples at once, take one to two hours, and cost about 25 ¢ per bottle of blood examined.

Possible Interfering Materials and Conditions. Interfering materials are not yet reported. Interfering conditions that may produce false positives in the donor blood include leukemia, Down's syndrome (mongolism), leprosy, and chronic renal disease, but patients with these conditions ought not be blood donors anyway.

Normal Range. Normally, the serum should be negative for hepatitis (Australia) antigen.

Heterophile Antibody

This is a test for infectious mononucleosis. In this disease, the level (titer) of antibodies to sheep erythrocytes rises for reasons that are not known. If the antibody level rises so that agglutination of sheep erythrocytes occurs at dilutions of 1:112 or greater, the test is considered positive. However, sometimes there are other anti-sheep erythrocyte antibodies in the blood, which are not related to infectious mononucleosis. Accordingly, it may be necessary to repeat the test by using more complicated techniques of antibody absorption.

Food and Drink Restrictions. None.

Procedure for Collecting Specimen. Venous blood is withdrawn, and 5 cc. placed in a test tube and allowed to coagulate. The test is performed on the serum.

A rapid slide test, suitable for office use, is now available also, and gives results in a few minutes.

Laboratory Procedure. Serial dilutions of the patient's serum are added to washed suspensions of sheep erythrocytes in a series of test tubes and incubated. The greatest dilution which agglutinates the erythrocytes is noted.

Possible Interfering Materials and Conditions. None reported yet.

Normal Range. Agglutination in concentrations up to 1:28.

Hinton

See Serological Tests for Syphilis

HLDH

See Heat Stable Lactic Dehydrogenase

I.B.C.

See Iron Binding Capacity

Icterus Index

This is a measure of the degree of yellowness of the serum. It is a simple way to determine whether there is excess bilirubin (bile pigment) in the serum. The test, however, cannot differentiate between bilirubin due to excess hemolysis, or due to obstruction of the biliary tract. The test is useful in discovering early jaundice not yet visible, or in following the course of frank jaundice.

Food and Drink Restrictions. None.

Procedure for Collecting Specimen. Venous blood is withdrawn and 5 cc. placed in a test tube and allowed to clot.

This test is performed on the serum.

Laboratory Procedure. The color of the serum is compared to the color of a standard solution of potassium bichromate, using a colorimeter.

Possible Interfering Materials and Conditions. The icterus index may be elevated if the patient has eaten large amounts of carrots. There is also a possibility that sweet potatoes might also elevate the icterus index.

Novobiocin and quinacrine (Atabrine) may also produce an apparent increase in icterus index.

Normal Range. 4 to 6 units.

I.I.

See Icterus Index

Immunoglobulins

See Plasma Electrophoresis for Gammopathies

Insulin Tolerance

This test is useful in differentiating between hypopituitarism and primary hypothyroidism. After injection of insulin in the former condition, the blood glucose level drops to about 50 per cent in 20 to 30 minutes. In the latter condition, the fall is less and requires at least 45 minutes. This test is of no value in the diagnosis of hyperinsulinism.

Food and Drink Restrictions. The patient must have been on an adequate diet for at least 3 days, and must fast for 12 hours before the test. Water is permitted.

Procedure for Collecting Specimen. Before proceeding with the test there must be on hand a concentrated glucose solution in a sterile syringe. This may be a lifesaving precaution.

A sample of venous blood is withdrawn and 3 cc. placed in a fluoride bottle. The doctor injects the insulin intravenously. Ordinarily the dose is 0.1 unit of regular insulin per kg. of body weight. However, if Addison's disease or adrenal insufficiency is suspected, the dose is less: 0.03 unit per kg. of body weight.

The patient is watched *continuously* for a possible sudden reaction. A physician should be within call to treat any severe reaction immediately with intravenous glucose. A reaction often begins with extreme nervousness, hunger, sweating and salivation. Disorders of speech and vision occur, and tremors and convulsions may be seen.

Venous blood samples (3 cc.) are collected 20, 30, 45, 60, 90 and 120 minutes after administration of insulin and placed in fluoride bottles or tubes. Care must be taken to label each blood sample with time of collection.

Laboratory Procedure. Same as described under *Glucose.*

Possible Interfering Materials and Conditions. None reported yet.

Normal Range. A return to the pre-injection level within 2 hours.

Iron

Small amounts of iron are carried in the serum, combined with the proteins. This iron is in balance with the iron concentration in the rest of the body, and variations in its levels can reflect disturbances in other areas of iron storage and utilization. In iron deficiency (microcytic) anemia, the serum iron levels will be lower than normal. The levels are higher than normal in hemolytic disorders, in untreated macrocytic anemias and in hemochromatosis (a condition of excess iron deposition in the liver and elsewhere).

Food and Drink Restrictions. None.

Procedure for Collecting Specimen. Special needles, syringes and procedures are needed. The amount of iron in the serum is very low—in the range of *micrograms* (millionths of a gram) per 100 ml. Ordinary needles and syringes may have enough traces of iron in them to give completely erroneous results. Hemolysis of the blood can also give false results. If a serum iron test is ordered, the clinical laboratory should be called for special needles, syringes and instructions. Ordinarily, 20 cc. of blood will be needed, and the test is done on the serum.

Laboratory Procedure. The iron is oxidized to the ferric state, and a thiocyanate solution added. The color reaction is then measured by a spectrophotometer.

Possible Interfering Materials and Conditions. A patient who has been anemic, and has recently begun to correct the anemia by more red blood cell production following the administration of cyanocobalamin (Vitamin B_{12}) or folic acid, may have low serum iron levels despite an adequate iron balance.

Hemolysis of the sample will produce a falsely elevated reading.

The serum iron level may be elevated by oral contraceptives.

Normal Range. 90 to 150 microgm. per 100 cc. of serum in males; 70 to 130 microgm. per 100 cc. of serum in females.

Iron-Binding Capacity (Unsaturated)

This test measures the amount of extra iron which could be carried in the plasma. Iron is transported in plasma by a protein, transferrin (also called siderophilin). Ordinarily, the actual serum iron is about 1/3 the level of the total iron-binding capacity. The measurement of unsaturated iron-binding capacity is particularly useful in the early diagnosis of hemochromatosis, a condition in which excess iron is deposited in vital tissues interfering with their function. If diagnosed early enough, suitable therapeutic measures can be most helpful. In hemochromatosis, the transferrin is highly saturated with iron, so that the unsaturated iron-binding capacity is quite low. There is also some lowering of unsaturated iron-binding capacity in pernicious anemia, hemolytic anemia, cirrhosis of the liver, uremia, and some infections. Unsaturated iron-binding capacity may be increased in iron deficiency anemia, in acute chronic blood loss, and in pregnancy.

Food and Drink Restrictions. None.

Procedure for Collecting Specimen. It is not clear whether or not special needles, syringes and procedures are necessary for this test. However, different types and makes of hypodermic needles may release different amounts of iron into specimens. Accordingly, the laboratory should be consulted before blood is drawn, and asked whether the regular hospital equipment is satisfactory for this test. Venous blood is drawn, and 10 cc. placed in a test tube and allowed to coagulate. The test is performed on serum, but it can also be done on plasma separated from uncoagulated blood if the anticoagulant used was heparin. Some laboratories use micro methods and can perform the test on a much smaller sample.

Laboratory Procedure. A known quantity of iron salt is added to the serum, and the amount which is not bound to transferrin is measured by means of a color reaction with a color reagent.

Possible Interfering Materials and Conditions. The iron-binding capacity may be elevated by oral contraceptives.

Hemolysis of the sample will make accurate readings impossible.

Normal Range. Since this test is a fairly recent one, there is still some disagreement about normal ranges. A reasonable estimate is 250 to 410 micrograms per 100 cc. of serum or plasma.

Kahn

See Serological Tests for Syphilis

Kolmer

See Serological Tests for Syphilis

Lactic Dehydrogenase

This test is used primarily as an aid in the diagnosis of myocardial infarction. Lactic dehydrogenases are enzymes found in serum and in several organs including the heart. Therefore, an increase in levels of lactic dehydrogenase is not specific, but in conjunction with other tests can help diagnose the presence of myocardial infarction. After an infarction occurs, the serum level of lactic dehydrogenase shows a perceptible rise in 6 to 12 hours, and may reach levels of from 2 to 10 times normal in 1 to 3 days. The elevated levels persist from 1 to 3 weeks after the infarction. There may also be markedly elevated levels in untreated acute leukemia, malignant lymphoma, megaloblastic anemia, sickle-cell anemia, liver disease, and extensive carcinomas. There is some disagreement about whether the levels are elevated in pulmonary infarction.

Food and Drink Restrictions. None.

Procedure for Collecting Specimen. Venous blood is withdrawn and 4 ml. placed in a test tube and allowed to coagulate. Hemolysis must be avoided. The red blood cells contain high levels of the enzyme, and if hemolysis occurs, high levels may be obtained as an artifact.

Laboratory Procedure. A sample of serum is added to pyruvic acid in the presence of diphosphopyridine nucleotide. The lactic dehydrogenase in the serum converts some of the pyruvic acid to lactic acid. The remaining pyruvic acid is measured with a color reagent in a spectrophotometer.

Possible Interfering Materials and Conditions. If any oxalate comes in contact with the specimen, it will cause falsely low readings.

Normal Range. 150-500 B & B units. There are other tests used to measure lactic dehydrogenase levels, and they use different types of units, in which normal range may be 30 to 120 units. Therefore, it is advisable to find out what your laboratory uses as the normal range.

Lactic Dehydrogenase, Heat Stable

See Heat Stable Lactic Dehydrogenase

Latex Slide Agglutination

This is primarily a test for rheumatoid arthritis. Empirically, it has been found that serum from patients with rheumatoid arthritis will cause small biologically inert particles, coated with human gamma globulin, to clump together. The usual type of biologically inert material employed is polystyrene latex. Like other tests for rheumatoid arthritis, this one is not specific. It is positive in other diseases of the connective tissues, such as lupus erythematosus and dermatomyositis, and in some chronic infections.

Food and Drink Restrictions. None.

Procedure for Collecting Specimen. Venous blood is withdrawn and 5 cc. placed in a test tube and allowed to coagulate. The test is performed on the serum.

Laboratory Procedure. A series of dilutions of the patient's serum is added to a suspension of polystyrene latex particles, coated with gamma globulin. The highest dilution of the serum producing agglutination is the end point.

Possible Interfering Materials and Conditions. None reported yet.

Normal Range. Agglutination up to and including the 1:40 dilution is normal.

L.D.

See Lactic Dehydrogenase

LDH

See Lactic Dehydrogenase

L.E.

See Lupus Erythematosus Cell Test

Lead

The usual use for this test is in suspected cases of acute lead poisoning, or an acute episode superimposed on chronic lead intoxication. This is a particularly important test in some areas of rundown housing in which children may eat peeling lead-based paint.

Food and Drink Restrictions. None.

Procedure for Collecting Specimen. Venous blood is withdrawn and 10 cc. placed in a test tube containing an anticoagulant. The test is performed on the whole blood.

Laboratory Procedure. Both chemical and spectrographic methods are available. The latter is based on the absorption by the lead of specific wavelengths of light.

Possible Interfering Materials and Conditions. None reported.

Normal Range. O to 5 mgm. per 100 ml. of whole blood.

Leucine Aminopeptidase

At one time an elevated serum level of the enzyme leucine aminopeptidase was thought to be specific for carcinoma of the pancreas. However, it has also been found to be elevated in a wide variety of diseases, including cirrhosis of the liver, viral hepatitis, infectious mononucleosis, stone in the common bile duct, acute pancreatitis, and acute cholecystitis. Furthermore, it has been shown that many patients with carcinoma of the pancreas have normal serum levels of leucine aminopeptidase. Therefore, the value of this test appears to be quite limited. Normal levels tend to make the diagnosis of carcinoma of the pancreas less likely, but do not rule it out.

Food and Drink Restrictions. None.

Procedure for Collecting Specimen. Venous blood is withdrawn, and 4 cc. placed in a test tube and allowed to coagulate. The test is performed on the serum.

Laboratory Procedure. A sample of serum is added to a peptide containing leucine, and beta-naphthylamine. The enzyme in the serum splits the peptide and the beta-naphthylamine produced reacts with a color reagent and is read by photometer.

Possible Interfering Materials and Conditions. None reported yet.

Normal Range. Varies with the method.

Male serum: 75 to 230 units per 100 cc.

Female serum: 80 to 210 units per 100 cc.

Leukocyte Count

See Blood Counts, White Cell Count

Lipase

This is a test for damage to the pancreas. Like amylase, lipase is secreted by the pancreas, and small amounts pass into the blood. In diseases such as acute pancreatitis and carcinoma of the pancreas, the blood level of lipase rises. Both amylase and lipase levels rise at the same rate, but the elevation in lipase concentration persists for a longer period. The lipase determination is, therefore, made when too much time has elapsed for the amylase level to remain elevated.

Food and Drink Restrictions. It is not clear whether or not the eating of food interferes with this test, since the test itself is not considered precise or completely accurate. It would probably be best, when practical, to draw the serum sample before breakfast after an overnight fast. If this cannot be done, a note should be made in the chart, indicating when the sample was drawn in relation to the last meal. Water may be taken freely.

Procedure for Collecting Specimen. Venous blood is withdrawn and 6 cc. placed in a test tube and allowed to coagulate. The test is performed on the serum.

Laboratory Procedure. The serum sample is incubated with an oil. The amount of fatty acid liberated is titrated.

Possible Interfering Materials and Conditions. Serum lipase levels may be elevated into a distinctly abnormal range if the patient has received bethanechol (Myocholine, Urecholine), codeine or morphine. Although definite evidence is not available, it seems prudent to assume that the other narcotic drugs may also produce falsely high levels of serum lipase if taken within the 24 hours before the sample is drawn.

Normal Range. Not over 1.5 units.

Lipid Fractions

This test measures the amounts of the several lipid

fractions in the serum. Lipids are substances that are chemically related to fatty acids. In certain diseases one or more lipid fraction concentrations are elevated. For example, in hypothyroidism, cholesterol is elevated; in nephrotic syndrome, total lipids are extremely high; in glycogen storage diseases and in ketosis, total lipids are elevated. There are, in addition, at least 5 types of primary, congenital types of hyperlipemia in which the lipids are carried bound to protein (hyperlipoproteinemias) that require additional tests for diagnosis. There is also substantial evidence that atherosclerosis is related to excess concentration of one or more lipid fractions in the serum, but the precise relationship is still unproven. Often a physician orders a measurement of lipid fractions in the hope that it will furnish a clue to the management of a patient with actual or suspected atherosclerosis.

Food and Drink Restrictions. The patient should be on a normal diet for 3 weeks before the test, and must fast for 12 hours before the blood sample is drawn. Water may be taken ad lib.

Procedure for Collecting Specimen. Venous blood is withdrawn and 20 cc. placed in test tubes and allowed to coagulate. The test is performed on the serum.

Laboratory Procedure. Each lipid fraction is measured by a different chemical procedure, all of them quite complex.

Possible Interfering Materials and Conditions. None reported yet.

Normal Range. There is considerable variation among laboratories:

Total lipids	400 to 800 mg./100 ml.
Phospholipids	150 to 380 mg./100 ml.
Cholesterol, total	120 to 260 mg./100 ml. (see also Cholesterol, P.60)
Cholesterol, free	Up to 50 mg./100 ml.
Cholesterol, esters	Up to 210 mg./100 ml.
Triglycerides (neutral fat)	25 to 150 mg./100 ml.
Free fatty acids	0.3 to 1.0 mEq./L.

Lipoprotein Analysis

This is a test to determine the presence or absence of certain disorders of fat metabolism. The lipids, which include fats and related compounds, are generally found in combination with one or more of the serum proteins. The combination of lipid and protein is called lipoprotein. At least 5 different types of familial disorder of lipid and lipoprotein metabolism are known. They are designated as I, II, III, IV, and V. Prognosis and management differ for each, and it is therefore helpful to know exactly which type of disorder a particular patient has. In addition, there may be other types of either familial or acquired lipoprotein disorder that have not yet been classified.

Food and Drink Restrictions. The patient should be on a normal diet for 3 weeks before the test, and must fast for 12 hours before the blood sample is drawn. Water may be taken ad lib.

Procedure for Collecting Specimen. Many institutions now use a micro method. Venous blood is withdrawn and 4 cc. placed in a test tube and allowed to coagulate. The test is performed on the serum.

Laboratory Procedure. The sample is subjected to electrophoresis, and the lipoprotein bands compared to standards.

Possible Interfering Materials and Conditions. None reported yet.

Normal Range. The normal range is determined by comparison with standard electrophoresis patterns.

Lithium

This test is used to monitor the lithium dosage in treatment of manic-depressive psychosis. Lithium, the lightest metal, forms salts that are similar to sodium salts. Once used as a sodium substitute in some diets, lithium salts were abandoned in the 1940's because their toxicity was too high when compared to the benefits. Then, in 1949, Dr. Cade in Australia found that lithium salts can correct the mania in manic depression, and it was also discovered that lithium can help prevent the depression. The seriousness of manic-depression is so great that the toxicity of lithium salts is not a contraindication to their use in this condition.

Ironically, because of poor coordination and information exchange among scientists, Cade's great discovery was ignored in this country for over 15 years, and only now are patients deriving benefit from it. The serum concentration of lithium must be kept within rather close limits to be effective and yet non-toxic. Therefore, patients receiving lithium salts must have serum levels checked regularly. The therapeutic level ranges from 0.6 to 1.6 milliequivalents per liter. At levels over 2.0 milliequivalents per liter, severe toxicity may occur, and dosage must be stopped or reduced.

Food and Drink Restrictions. None reported, but there are restrictions on intake of medication (see *Normal Range,* below).

Procedure for Collecting Specimen. The patient must not have taken any lithium in the preceding 8 hours. Venous blood is withdrawn and 6 cc. placed in a plain glass tube and allowed to clot.

Laboratory Procedure. The serum concentration of lithium is measured in a flame photometer.

Possible Interfering Materials and Conditions. None reported yet.

Normal Range. Normally, there are no measurable lithium levels in the serum. The *therapeutic* levels in patients treated with lithium are 0.6 to 1.6 mEq. per liter. (Some authorities use 1.5 mEq. per liter as the upper limit.)

Lupus Erythematosus (L.E.) Cell Test

A particular type of cell called the lupus erythematosus cell, is often seen in lupus erythematosus. Finding this cell can help in the diagnosis, although it may also be found in other conditions.

Food and Drink Restrictions. None.

Procedure for Collecting Specimen. The exact method to be used depends on the laboratory. In a common method, venous blood is withdrawn and 5 cc. placed in an oxalate bottle or tube. In another method, 7 cc. of blood are placed in a tube without an anticoagulant, and the laboratory performs the test on the clot.

Laboratory Procedure. The leucocytes of the blood are concentrated by centrifugation, smeared and stained. The stained smears are then examined microscopically.

Possible Interfering Materials and Conditions. None reported yet.

Normal Range. Normally there are no lupus erythematosus cells.

Magnesium

In magnesium deficiency, a state of tetany can sometimes occur, which in appearance is indistinguishable from the tetany of low calcium. Accordingly, in tetanic or pre-tetanic conditions, serum magnesium levels may be measured to see if they are abnormally low. If they are, magnesium salts usually correct the symptoms. In patients receiving large amounts of parenteral fluids for long periods, serum magnesium levels may be measured in an attempt to diagnose an early magnesium deficiency and correct it before tetany occurs.

Food and Drink Restrictions. None.

Procedure for Collecting Specimen. Venous blood is withdrawn, and 5 cc. placed in a test tube and allowed to coagulate. The test is performed on the serum. At times, this test may be designated "emergency" by the physician.

Laboratory Procedure. There are several methods available for determination of magnesium levels. It appears as if the measurement by flame photometer is likely to become most common.

Possible Interfering Materials and Conditions. None reported yet.

Normal Range.
1.7 to 2.8 mgm. per 100 cc. of serum, or
1.5 to 2.3 milliequivalents per liter.

Malaria Film

This is a test for malaria parasites in the blood. It is important not only is establishing a definite diagnosis of malaria but also in determining which species of malarial parasite is involved. Each species can be identified on the film.

Food and Drink Restrictions. None.

Procedure for Performing Test and Collecting Specimen. A film of blood is placed on a slide and stained with Giemsa stain. Depending on the number of parasites, a thin or thick film of blood may be best. The slides are examined microscopically for parasites.

If the first films are negative, they should be repeated 6 to 12 hours after a chill, when there is a greater likelihood of finding the parasites in the blood.

Possible Interfering Materials and Conditions. None reported yet.

Normal Range. Normally there are no malaria parasites in the blood.

Mazzini

See Serological Tests for Syphilis

Methemoglobin

Methemoglobin is not ordinarily present in the blood. It is found when the hemoglobin is oxidized by chemicals such as nitrites, chlorates, etc. Drinking well water containing nitrites is a frequent cause of methemoglobinemia. Methemoglobin is not an oxygen carrier like hemoglobin.

Food and Drink Restrictions. None.

Procedure for Collecting Specimen. Venous blood is withdrawn and 5 cc. placed in an oxalate tube or bottle. Another acceptable anticoagulant is sodium citrate.

Laboratory Procedure. Methemoglobin is detected by the use of the spectroscope which shows the absorption bands of this substance when light is passed through it.

Possible Interfering Materials and Conditions. None reported yet.

Normal Range. Normally there is no methemoglobin in the blood.

Non-Protein Nitrogen (N.P.N.)

This is a general test of kidney function. It is not as sensitive as certain other tests and cannot be used to discover early kidney disease. About half of the non-protein nitrogen is usually urea, which is normally excreted by the kidney. The remainder consists of amino acids, ammonia, creatine, creatinine, uric acid, and some unidentified substances. When kidney function is markedly diminished the urea, and, therefore, the non-protein nitrogen level in the blood, rises. This measurement is less accurate than the urea nitrogen test. There is no reason to do both tests.

Food and Drink Restrictions. None.

Procedure for Collecting Specimen. Venous blood is withdrawn, and 5 cc. placed in an oxalate tube or bottle. EDTA should *not* be used as an anticoagulant since it produces a spurious elevation of N.P.N.

Laboratory Procedure. The nitrogenous substances are converted to ammonia which is then measured by titration.

Possible Interfering Materials and Conditions. EDTA in the specimen container will give a spurious elevation of the N.P.N.

Normal Range. 15 to 35 mg. per 100 cc. of serum.

N.P.N.

See Non-Protein Nitrogen

OGTT

See Glucose Tolerance

Partial Thromboplastin Time (PTT)

This has become a widely used screening test for blood coagulation in general. It is considered more sensitive than

the clotting (coagulation) time test. The partial thromboplastin time is elevated in most types of clotting disorders,
but not in deficiences of Factor VII or platelets. If the test
results are abnormal, additional tests are performed to
determine the precise kind of defect that exists.

Food and Drink Restrictions. None.

Procedure for Collecting Specimen. Variations in procedure are reported, with some authorities recommending
a two-syringe technique, and others recommending the
usual technique which is described here. Venous blood is
withdrawn, and exactly 4.5 ml. placed in a special tube
containing a special sodium oxalate solution. Ordinary oxalate
bottles cannot be used. Alternately, a special vacutainer
specifically for this test may be used.

Laboratory Procedure. The sample is centrifuged to
obtain plasma to which is added, at constant temperature
conditions, partial thromboplastin suspension and calcium
chloride. The time taken to produce a fibrin clot is measured
by a stopwatch. Some laboratories use modifications of the
basic procedure to try to get greater specificity and uni-
formity. Such modifications can sometimes alter the normal
range. The results should always be compared to a standard
run at the same time.

Possible Interfering Materials and Conditions. If a vacuum tube used to collect the specimen is not completely
filled, the partial thromboplastin time may be spuriously
elevated because of the effect of extra anticoagulant in the
tube.

Normal Range. The normal range varies in different
laboratories, depending on the source of some of the
reagents used. Ordinarily, the partial thromboplastin time
is 60 to 70 seconds, but some laboratories consider 100
seconds as the upper limit of normal. Comparison with the
control time as determined on a standardized sample of
plasma may be a more accurate measure of normality. Partial
thromboplastin times within 5 seconds of the control time
are normal; those 6 to 10 seconds longer than the control

time are equivocal; those 11 to 20 seconds longer than the control time are probably abnormal; and those over 20 seconds longer than the control time are definitely abnormal.

Paul-Bunnell Test

See Heterophile Antibody

P.B.I.

See Protein-Bound Iodine

Partial Pressure of Carbon Dioxide (Pco$_2$)

This is a measure of the partial pressure of carbon dioxide in a gas phase in equilibrium with blood. It is usually measured on arterial blood, although deep capillary blood is sometimes used. Levels of arterial Pco$_2$ above normal may stem from a congenital cardiovascular defect, interference with respiratory exchange, or various lung disorders. Interpretation of the significance of abnormal Pco$_2$ levels, therefore, depends on correlation with clinical findings and with the Po$_2$ (partial pressure of oxygen) and pH. The physician may designate this test "emergency."

Food and Drink Restrictions. None reported.

Procedure for Collecting Specimen. The patient should be at rest for at least 15 minutes. The sample of arterial blood is collected by a physician, preferably in a heparinized vacutainer tube. The tube should be completely filled with blood.

Laboratory Procedure. The Pco$_2$ is measured directly on an electronic meter consisting of a pH meter adapted for Pco$_2$ measurements.

Possible Interfering Materials and Conditions. None reported.

Normal Range. Normally, the *arterial* Pco$_2$ is 31 to 45 mm. of mercury.

P.C.V. (Packed Cell Volume)

See Hematocrit

pH

This is a measure of acidity or alkalinity. The normal blood pH ranges from 7.35 to 7.45. The pH may be lower in such conditions as hypoventilation, severe diarrhea, Addison's disease, and diabetic acidosis. The pH may rise above normal levels in conditions such as excess vomiting, Cushing's syndrome, and hyperventilation.

Food and Drink Restrictions. None.

Procedure for Collecting Specimen. Venous blood should be withdrawn without using a tourniquet, if possible. If a tourniquet is necessary, the patient should *not* open and close his fist, but should keep it closed without straining. For years, the blood sample was collected under oil. However, there is a growing trend away from oil. Instead, vacuum tubes containing heparin are used, and 5 cc. of blood collected in them. In some hospitals, oiled syringes are still used, and can give satisfactory results. If an anticoagulant is used, it should be heparin.

Laboratory Procedure. A sensitive pH-meter measures the pH electronically.

Possible Interfering Materials and Conditions. None reported yet.

Normal Range. pH 7.35 to 7.45.

Phenylketonuria

See Guthrie

Phosphatase, Acid

This is a test to identify metastasizing carcinomas of the prostate. Normally, small amounts of acid phosphatase are found in the serum. The prostate gland is exceptionally rich in this enzyme and so are carcinomas of the prostate. The normal gland and the carcinoma which has not yet spread do not release the enzyme into the serum. However, the metastasizing prostate carcinoma does, increasing the serum concentration markedly. The test is performed only on men. Other conditions besides carcinoma of the prostate which produce elevated serum acid phosphatase levels include: Paget's disease, hyperparathyroidism, metastatic mammary carcinoma, multiple myeloma, some liver diseases, renal insufficiency, osteogenesis imperfecta, thrombocytosis, arterial embolism, myocardial infarction, thrombophlebitis, pulmonary embolism, and sickle-cell crisis.

Food and Drink Restrictions. None.

Procedure for Collecting Specimen. Venous blood is removed and 2.5 cc. placed in each of 2 test tubes (total 5 cc.) and allowed to clot. The test is performed on the serum.

Laboratory Procedure. The speed with which a sample of serum hydrolyzes a monophosphate ester at pH 5 is measured.

Possible Interfering Materials and Conditions. If the patient has had a prostatic massage, or extensive palpation of the prostate, there may be elevation of the serum acid phosphatase to abnormal levels for about 24 hours.

Hemolysis of the specimen can produce spuriously high levels.

The following may give spurious elevations of acid phosphatase levels:

Atromid
°Clofibrate

The following may give spurious decrease of acid phosphatase levels:

Fluorides
Oxalates
Phosphates

Normal Range:
Up to 4 King-Armstrong units, or
Up to 1.1 Bodansky units, or
Up to .63 Bessey-Lowry units.

Phosphatase, Alkaline

This test may be used in the diagnosis of bone as well as

of liver diseases. Normally, there is a small amount of alkaline phosphatase in the serum. In bone diseases, however, the alkaline phosphatase rises in proportion to the formation of new bone cells. This test, therefore, may be of value in differentiating between various bone disorders, including tumors. In disorders of the liver and biliary tract, the alkaline phosphatase rises because excretion is impaired. This test may therefore also be of some use in evaluating the degree of blockage of the biliary tract.

The alkaline phosphatase levels are elevated in hyperparathyroidism, osteitis deformans, osteomalacia, Goucher's disease, rickets, healing fractures, Boeck's sarcoid, hyperthyroidism (Grave's disease), leukemia, after administration of large amounts of vitamin D, and in pregnancy.

Food and Drink Restrictions. None.

Procedure for Collecting Specimen. Venous blood is withdrawn and 2.5 cc. placed in each of 2 test tubes (total 5 cc.) and allowed to clot. The test is performed on the serum.

Laboratory Procedure. The speed with which a sample of serum hydrolyzes a phosphate ester at pH 9.7 is measured.

Possible Interfering Materials and Conditions. The alkaline phosphatase levels may be elevated by several drugs. In some cases, the elevation results from an action of the drug on body enzymes, but the increased level does not indicate bone or liver disease. Because the number of drugs that cause elevation of alkaline phosphatase levels is large, only official (generic) names are listed:

Acetohexamide	Lincomycin
Allopurinol	Methyldopa
Anabolic agents, some	Oral contraceptives, some
Androgens, some	Oxacillin
Chlorpropamide	Penicillamine
Colchicine	Phenothiazines, some
Erythromycin	Procainamide
Gold salts	Thiothixene
n-Hydroxyacetamide	Tolazamide
Indomethacin	Tolbutamide

Large amounts of Vitamin D can also produce elevations in the serum level of alkaline phosphatase.

Normal Range:	Adults	Children
King-Armstrong units	4 to 13	15 to 30
Bodansky units	1.5 to 4.5	5 to 14
Bessy-Lowry units	.8 to 2.3	2.8 to 6.7

Phosphorus (Inorganic)

Phosphorus metabolism is directly associated with calcium metabolism and involves many organs and physiological functions. The concentration of phosphorus may be increased in severe kidney disease, hypoparathyroidism, acromegaly, or excessive vitamin D intake. The concentration may decrease in rickets, hyperparathyroidism, and certain diseases of the kidney tubules.

Food and Drink Restrictions. None.

Procedure for Collecting Specimen. Venous blood is withdrawn and 4 cc. placed in a test tube and allowed to coagulate. The test is performed on the serum.

Laboratory Procedure. A protein-free sample of the serum is added to the standard reagents which produce a blue color. The intensity of the color is then measured with a colorimeter.

Possible Interfering Materials and Conditions. The phosphorus level may be elevated if the patient has received diphenylhydantoin (Dilantin), heparin, pituitrin, or vitamin D. It may be interfered with or increased if the patient has received epinephrine (Adrenalin) or insulin.

Normal Range:
Adults, 3.0 to 4.5 mg. per 100 cc. of serum;
children, 4.0 to 6.5 mg. per 100 cc. of serum.

Platelet Count

See Blood Counts, Platelet Count

Plasma Electrophoresis for Gammopathies

This is a test for abnormalities in the gamma globulin fraction of the plasma. Plasma proteins are divided into albumins, globulins, and fibrinogens. The globulins, in turn are divided into alpha, beta, and gamma globulins, depending on their electrophoresis pattern. The gamma globulins are themselves divided into 5 major groups, G, A, M, D, L. The gamma globulins include most of the antibodies that fight infections, and a disorder involving these gamma globulins may result in increased susceptibility to infection. Such disorders may be inherited, or they may be associated with some neoplasms, and with some infections. The term "immunoglobulins," abbreviated Ig, is now supplanting the term gamma globulins.

Food and Drink Restrictions. None reported yet.

Procedure for Collecting Specimen. Venous blood is withdrawn and 5 cc. placed in a test tube and allowed to coagulate.

Laboratory Procedure. A sample of serum is subjected to electrophoresis and the pattern produced is compared to standard patterns.

Possible Interfering Materials and Conditions. Recent transfusions of blood or plasma, or administration of antisera might produce spurious results.

Normal Range. The normal range is determined by reference to standard electrophoresis patterns.

Po_2

This is a measure of the partial pressure of oxygen in a gas phase in equilibrium with blood. It is usually measured on arterial blood, although deep capillary blood is sometimes used. Levels of Po_2 below normal may stem from a variety of conditions such as congenital heart defects, interference with respiratory exchange, and a variety of lung disorders. Interpretation of the significance of abnormal Po_2 levels therefore depends on correlation with clinical findings and with the P_{CO_2} and pH. The physician may designate this test "emergency."

Food and Drink Restrictions. None reported.

Procedure for Collecting Specimen. The patient should be at rest for at least 15 minutes before the sample of arterial blood is collected by a physician, preferably in a heparinized vacutainer tube. The tube should be completely filled with blood.

Laboratory Procedure. The P_{O_2} is measured directly on an electronic meter consisting of a pH meter adapted for P_{O_2} measurements.

Possible Interfering Materials and Conditions. None reported yet.

Normal Range. Normally, the *arterial* P_{O_2} is 75 to 95 mm. of mercury.

Potassium

Potassium is an essential ion found in large concentrations in all cells and in much smaller concentrations in the serum. Alterations in serum potassium levels may produce serious changes in body function, or even death. A marked decrease in serum potassium may cause cardiac arrhythmias and muscle weakness; a marked increase produces a series of electrocardiographic changes and arrhythmias. There may also be depression, lethargy, and coma. Therefore, when it is suspected that serum potassium levels have changed, tests should be made and measures taken to restore them to the normal range. Increased serum potassium levels may be found in conditions of severe cell damage and destruction, adrenal cortical deficiency, and hypoventilation. A decrease in serum potassium may be found in severe diarrhea, periodic familial paralysis, chronic kidney disease, excess function of the adrenal cortex, and following administration of insulin and glucose in diabetes without added potassium. Low serum potassium levels are particularly dangerous when digitalis glycosides are being administered.

It has been reported that low serum potassium levels

in the presence of hypertension suggests primary aldoster-
onism.

Food and Drink Restrictions. None.

Procedure for Collecting Specimen. Venous blood is withdrawn, preferably with a special oiled syringe and 6 cc. placed
in a test tube under oil. The oil is used to minimize friction
and the resulting hemolysis of red cells. In many institutions,
a plain tube is used for collection of the blood.

Laboratory Procedure. The serum concentration of potassium is measured in a flame photometer.

Possible Interfering Materials and Conditions. The serum
potassium level may be elevated by tobacco smoke. It may
be decreased by several drugs. However, this decrease is a
true decrease in the actual potassium level, and not a spurious
or misleading effect on a test procedure. The fact that these
drugs have such effects cannot be considered as interference
with test results; indeed many times the test is ordered by
the doctor precisely because he wishes to know the extent to
which a prescribed drug is affecting serum potassium levels.
The materials having such an effect include acetazolamide,
ACTH, cortisone and some of its derivatives, P-aminosalicylic
acid, and glucose.

Normal Range:
4 to 5 milliequivalents per liter, or
16 to 22 mg. per 100 cc. of serum.

Protein-Bound Iodine (P.B.I.)

This is a test of thyroid function. The thyroid gland binds
iodine to organic compounds, mainly the hormone thyroxin.
This hormone is precipitated by chemicals which precipitate
proteins, so that a measurement of the amount of iodine in
a protein precipitate indicates the amount of thyroid hormone present. An increased concentration of protein-bound
iodine is usually found in hyperthyroidism, although it may
also be seen in early hepatitis. A decreased concentration of
protein-bound iodine is usually found in hypothyroidism.

Food and Drink Restrictions. None.

Procedure for Collecting Specimen. The patient must not have received any iodine-containing drugs nor any iodine-containing contrast media for the appropriate period before performing this test. (See table 22.) Venous blood is withdrawn and 8 cc. placed in a test tube and allowed to coagulate. The test is performed on the serum.

Laboratory Procedure. A protein precipitant is added to a sample of serum and the precipitate removed, washed, treated with alkali, and redissolved. Its ability to decolorize a yellow solution of ceric sulfate indicates the iodine content.

Possible Interfering Materials and Conditions. The protein-bound iodine levels are affected by so many medications that special efforts should be made to see that the patient does not take medications or receive radiographic contrast media for several days before the test. Unfortunately, some radiographic contrast media can produce false high results for long periods. In general, it should be assumed that all radiopaque, iodine-containing injectable contrast media are likely to produce falsely elevated protein-bound iodine levels for 6 months. Some of these contrast media are believed to exert an effect for 20 or more years. The number of drugs affecting protein-bound iodine levels is so extensive that a listing of many of the brand names is not feasible. Accordingly, only official names will be presented.

The drugs which can produce a misleading *elevation* of the protein bound-iodine include:

Barbiturates (see table 18)
Barium sulfate (use in GI
  series and barium enema)
Estrogens (see table 21)
Gargles, some
Iodine-containing drugs
  (see table 22)
Lithium carbonate capsule
  dye
Metrecal
Mouth washes, some
Oral contraceptives
Perphenazine
Sun-tan lotions, some

The protein-bound iodine may be spuriously elevated if a patient has had intravenous solutions given by catheter before the sample is drawn. Iodine is leeched out of the catheter in amounts sufficient to alter test results.

In biliary tract obstruction, there may be a spurious elevation of the protein-bound iodine.

The drugs which can produce misleading *depression* of protein-bound iodine levels include:

ACTH
Androgens (see table 16)
Cortisone-like drugs (see table 20)
Diphenylhydantoin
Disulfiram
Gold salts (for weeks or months)
Isoniazid
Liothyronine
Mercurial diuretics
Para-aminobenzoic acid
Para-aminosalicylic acid
Phenothiazines except perphenazine
Phenylbutazone
Reserpine
Salicylates including aspirin (see table 27)
Sulfonamides
Thiazides
Thiocyanates
Tri-iodothyronine
Vitamin preparations, some

In addition, the Bromsulphalein retention test (B.S.P.) may produce false elevations or depressions of the protein-bound iodine levels.

Normal Range: 3.0 to 8.0 microgm. per 100 cc. of serum.

Protein, Total

See Albumin, Globulin, Total Protein, A/G Ratio

Prothrombin Time

This is an indirect test of the clotting ability of the blood. Prothrombin is converted to thrombin in the clotting process. When the prothrombin level of the blood is lower than normal, it is believed that the clotting tendency of the blood within the blood vessels is diminished. The prothrombin content of the blood is lowered in liver diseases, hypoprothrombinemia of infants, vitamin K deficiency, and following drug therapy. The vast majority of cases of low blood prothrombin results from the administration of Dicumarol or similar drugs. The substances are given to reduce the clotting tendency of the blood and thus avoid thromboembolic phenomena.

This test is often done daily during the acute stages of myocardial infarction, and accurate results are needed promptly in order to enable the physician to determine the size of the next dose of anticoagulant.

Food and Drink Restrictions. None.

Procedure for Collecting Specimen. Venous blood is withdrawn and exactly 4.5 cc. placed in a special test tube containing a special sodium oxalate solution, and mixed thoroughly. Ordinary oxalate bottles cannot be used.

Laboratory Procedure. There are several methods. The most commonly used is the one-stage method of Quick where a mixture of thromboplastin and calcium is added to the oxalated serum. The time of formation of fibrin threads is measured with a stop-watch. This result is then compared to that obtained on normal blood.

Possible Interfering Materials and Conditions. The prothrombin time may be falsely elevated by barbiturates (see table 18).

If the vacuum tube used to collect the specimen is not completely filled, the prothrombin time may be spuriously elevated because of the effect of extra anticoagulant in the tube.

The prothrombin time may be reduced by several groups of drugs, but it is not yet clear whether the reduction is an interference with a laboratory test, or whether it represents a true reduction in prothrombin levels via a biochemical effect on physiological functions, or on indigenous bacteria. The drugs which may reduce the prothrombin time include:

Antibiotics
Hydroxyzine (Vistaril)
Salicylates, including aspirin (see table 27)
Sulfonamides

Normal Range. Between 11 and 18 seconds, depending on type of thromboplastin used, is considered 100 per cent of normal. In Dicumarol treatment the physician tries to keep the prothrombin time at 2 to 2½ times normal. Expressed as prothrombin percentage, which is not a straight-line function of prothrombin time, a range of from 20 to 30 per cent is sought.

P.T.

See Prothrombin Time

P.T.T.

See Partial Thromboplastin Time

Red Cell Count

See Blood Counts, Red Cell Count

Red Cell Fragility

This is a test of the ability of the red blood cells to resist hemolysis in a hypotonic solution. As the concentration of salts outside the cell decreases, more water continues to pass into the cell by osmosis, and the membrane finally bursts. The salt concentration at which hemolysis occurs is taken as a measure of red blood cell fragility. Fragility is increased in congenital hemolytic jaundice and aplastic anemia.

Food and Drink Restrictions. None.

Procedure for Collecting Specimen. Venous blood is withdrawn into a completely dry syringe and 5 cc. placed in an oxalate bottle. For control purposes a similar 5 cc. sample is drawn from a normal person and placed in another oxalate bottle labeled "control."

Laboratory Procedure. Samples of the blood are added to solutions of sodium chloride varying in concentration from 0.28% to 0.6%, by steps of 0.02%. After gentle mixing, the mixtures are allowed to stand for several hours. The presence of hemolysis is shown by a clear red coloration of the supernatant plasma.

Possible Interfering Materials and Conditions. None reported yet.

Normal Range:
Slight hemolysis between 0.40 % and 0.46 % sodium chloride; complete hemolysis between 0.30 % and 0.36 % sodium chloride.

Reticulocyte Count
See Blood Counts, Reticulocyte Count

Rh Factor
See Blood Types, Rh Factor

Salicylates

Salicylate levels may be measured in two distinct types of situations. In some cases of rheumatic fever, large doses of salicylates are used to control symptoms. The blood level of the drug may be measured in an attempt to adjust dosage more effectively. It is generally considered necessary to have blood levels of at least 25 mgm. per 100 cc. for full therapeutic effect. Unfortunately, this level may be toxic to some children.

In cases of accidental poisoning, blood salicylate levels may be helpful in making correct decisions as to management. Salicylates (primarily aspirin) are the main causes of poisoning in children. In most cases, blood levels over 35 mgm. per 100 cc. are toxic.

Food and Drink Restrictions. None.

Procedure for Collecting Specimen. Venous blood is withdrawn and 5 cc. placed in a test tube and allowed to coagulate. The test is usually performed on the serum. It can also be done on plasma or blood which has been treated with any standard anticoagulant.

Laboratory Procedure. The sample is added to a reagent containing ferric ion which produces a purple color with salicylates. The concentration can be measured by colorimeter or spectrophotometer.

Possible Interfering Materials and Conditions. None reported yet.

Normal Range. Normally, there is no salicylate in the blood.

Sedimentation Rate

This test measures the rate at which red cells settle to the bottom of a glass test tube. The sedimentation rate is increased in infections and in conditions in which cell destruction occurs. This test is useful in diagnosing and following the course of such illnesses as rheumatic fever, arthritis and myocardial infarction.

Food and Drink Restrictions. None.

Procedure for Collecting Specimen. Venous blood is withdrawn and 4 cc. placed in an oxalate bottle.

Laboratory Procedure. A sample of the blood is placed in a special thin glass tube which is kept upright. The rate at which the upper part of the red cell column descends is measured and is usually reported as millimeters fall in 1 hour. Corrections for anemia are sometimes made and reported as "corrected" sedimentation rate.

Possible Interfering Materials and Conditions. None reported yet.

Normal Range. This depends to some extent on the type of glass tube used. In the Westergren method, which is common, the normal values for men are 0 to 15 mm. per hour and for women 0 to 20 mm. per hour.

Serological Tests (General)

These tests are used to identify substances in the serum which result from exposure to certain microorganisms. Often, the substance to be identified and quantitated is an antibody to the microorganism itself. An example is the Widal test for typhoid antibodies. Sometimes, the material of interest is an antibody to some enzyme elaborated by a microorganism, for example, antistreptolysin O. In many cases, however, the exact relationship between the microorganism and the serological material is unknown. Years of observation have shown that, in the presence of a particular disease, the body elaborates a substance which is readily measured. For example, in infectious mononucleosis, the body produces larger amounts than usual of antibodies to sheep red blood cells (*see Heterophile Antibody*). Similarly, we do not understand the relationship of the serological tests for syphilis to the Treponema which causes the disease.

Food and Drink Restrictions. None.

Procedure for Collecting Specimen. Venous blood is withdrawn and 5 cc. placed in a test tube and allowed to coagulate. The test is performed on the serum.

Laboratory Procedure. This varies with the type of test.

Possible Interfering Materials and Conditions. None reported yet.

Normal Range. There may be weak positive reactions to some serological tests in the absence of disease.

Serological Tests for Syphilis

There are several varieties, including the Wassermann, Kolmer, Kahn, Hinton, Mazzini and V.D.R.L. (Venereal Disease Research Laboratory) tests. All are nonspecific in nature and sometimes they are positive in diseases other than syphilis. Interpretation of these serological tests usually requires considerable skill and experience, as well as correlation with the clinical findings and history. In early primary syphilis the serology is negative. In late, adequately treated syphilis, the serology may be fixed at a high positive titer although the patient is, in effect, cured. In late, improperly treated syphilis, the serology may be negative even though the patient is not cured and is developing central nervous system involvement.

Serological tests for syphilis are performed routinely in many situations, often because of legal requirements. For example, many states require a serological test before marriage. Most physicians have these tests performed on all pregnant women to avoid congenital syphilis in the newborn. Many hospitals require a routine serology on all patients on admission.

Food and Drink Restrictions. None.

Procedure for Collecting Specimen. Venous blood is withdrawn and 5 cc. placed in a test tube and allowed to coagulate. The test is performed on the serum.

Laboratory Procedure. This varies with the test being performed.

Possible Interfering Materials and Conditions. In several diseases of the immune system, such as lupus erythematosus, there may be false positive serological tests for syphilis.

There may be a false positive VDRL test if cetylcide, a disinfectant, comes in contact with the specimen.

Normal Range. Normally these tests are negative. If the reaction is faintly positive, it may denote some disorder other than syphilis.

Serum Albumin . . . Serum Globulin . . . Serum Protein

See Albumin, Globulin, Total Protein, A/G Ratio

Serum hepatitis test

See Hepatitis Test

Serum Transaminase

Transaminases are enzymes which catalyze the transfer of an amino grouping (NH_2) from an amino acid to an alpha keto acid. There are several different kinds of transaminases. The most commonly measured ones are the glutamic oxaloacetic transaminase (sometimes abbreviated SGOT) and the glutamic pyruvic transaminase (sometimes abbreviated SGPT). Transaminases are found normally in heart, liver, muscle, kidney, and pancreas. Elevated serum levels are seen in disease conditions in which the transaminases leak from the dead or damaged cells into the serum. Since there are several transaminases in each type of cell, there are likely to be serum elevations of more than 1 type of transaminase when an organ is damaged. Accordingly, there is nothing specific about elevations of serum transaminase levels. Their value in diagnosis depends on careful comparison with the results of physical examinations and other laboratory tests.

Serum Glutamic Oxaloacetic Transaminase (SGOT)

In myocardial infarction, the GOT in the heart muscle cells leaks out and increases serum levels from 4 to 10 times. The peak level is usually reached about 24 hours after infarction, and returns to normal by about the fifth day. The test is used primarily in the diagnosis of myocardial infarction.

In liver diseases, serum GOT levels may be 10 to 100 times normal, and remain elevated for long periods. In the diagnosis and management of some types of liver disease, such as viral hepatitis, the level of serum GOT may provide useful information on the progress of the condition.

Food and Drink Restrictions. None.

Procedure for Collecting Specimen. Venous blood is withdrawn and 5 cc. placed in a test tube and allowed to coagulate. The test is performed on the serum. It is best to draw the blood before any drugs are given, even if at night. The enzyme is stable for about 4 days in the serum at refrigerator temperatures, so that a specimen can be drawn at any time, allowed to clot, and then placed in the refrigerator until the laboratory can test it. The time of withdrawing the blood should be noted.

Laboratory Procedure. There are several methods for measuring serum GOT. Currently, both colorimetric and spectrophotometric measurements are in use.

Possible Interfering Materials and Conditions. The drugs listed below can cause elevations in serum GOT levels. However, it is not yet clear whether the elevations are artifacts, or whether they result from slight liver damage by the drugs which are listed here by official (generic) names only:

Ampicillin
Azaserine
Carbenicillin
Chlorpromaine (Information on derivatives not
yet available)
Codeine
Dicumarol
Erythromycin
Ethyl biscoumacetate

Iproniazid	Pyrazinamide
Methyldopa	Pyridoxin
Morphine	Salicylates (see table 27)
Narcotics	Sulfamethoxypyridazine
Oxacillin	Vitamin B₆
Para-aminosalicylic acid	

The ingestion of lead, even without evident poisoning, may produce elevations to 300 to 400 units.

Normal Range. 10 to 40 units.

Serum Glutamic Pyruvic Transaminase (SGPT)

This enzyme, like the GOT, is found in several tissues, and its serum levels become elevated when these tissues are diseased. The serum GPT levels are used mainly in the diagnosis of liver disease. In cases of hepatitis, serum GPT rises higher than GOT levels, reaching levels of 4000 units. It falls slowly, reaching normal levels in about 2 to 3 months, unless complications occur. In cases of liver damage due to drugs and chemicals, the serum GPT levels can be even higher than in hepatitis. The major clinical value of the test appears to be in the differential diagnosis of jaundice. If the jaundice is caused by disease in the liver itself, serum GPT levels are likely to be considerably higher than 300 units. However, if the jaundice results from a condition outside the liver, the serum GPT levels are likely to be less than 300 units. In some cases comparison of serum GOT and GPT levels can give useful clues to the diagnosis, but the details of such comparisons are beyond the scope of this book.

Food and Drink Restrictions. None.

Procedure for Collecting Specimen. Venous blood is withdrawn and 5 cc. placed in a test tube and allowed to coagulate. The test is performed on the serum.

Laboratory Procedure. There are several methods for determining serum GPT. Currently, both colorimetric and spectrophotometric measurements are in use.

Possible Interfering Materials and Conditions. A number

of drugs and chemicals produce elevated serum GPT levels, but it appears that this is not an artifact, but the result of toxicity affecting the liver.

The ingestion of lead, even without evident poisoning, may produce elevations to 300 to 400 units.

Normal Range. 5 to 40 units.

S.G.O.T.

See Serum Transaminase

S.G.P.T.

See Serum Transaminase

SH Antigen

See Hepatitis Test

Sickle Cell Test

This test is performed to demonstrate an unusual type of red blood cell, containing a different type of hemoglobin which is relatively insoluble when unoxygenated. When the available oxygen is reduced the hemoglobin may precipitate within the cell, causing it to assume the shape of a sickle. This may interfere with the free flow of blood and cause various disorders. Most people with the sickling trait in their red cells have no demonstrable disease but may require special care and attention in surgery and obstetrics to avoid hypoxia (diminution of oxygen supply). Although the sickling trait is more often found in Negroes, it may also be found in other persons.

Food and Drink Restrictions. None.

Procedure for Performing Test and Collecting Specimen. There are several methods; the simplest employs a solution of sodium bisulfite in water. A drop of the solution is added to a drop of blood and the blood examined microscopically for the sickle-shaped cells.

Possible Interfering Materials and Conditions. If the

patient has received a blood transfusion within three months of the test, the results may be altered by the presence of the donor's red cells.

Normal Range. Sickling is not a disease in the usual sense. There is no normal or abnormal range.

Sodium

Sodium is the main cation of the blood and extracellular fluid. Its concentration may vary within narrow limits, but if these are exceeded, serious disturbances or even death may result. Increased serum sodium levels may be found in markedly inadequate water intake and following adminstration of excessive amounts of sodium. Decreased sodium levels may occur in diarrhea, heat exhaustion, Addison's disease and certain kidney disorders.

Food and Drink Restrictions. None.

Procedure for Collecting Specimen. Venous blood is withdrawn, preferably with a special oiled syringe and 6 cc. placed in a test tube under oil. The oil is used to minimize friction and the resulting hemolysis of red blood cells.

In many institutions, a plain tube is used for collection of the blood.

Laboratory Procedure. The serum concentration of sodium is measured in a flame photometer.

Possible Interfering Materials and Conditions. None reported yet.

Normal Range:
138 to 145 milliequivalents per liter, or
315 to 335 mg. per 100 cc. of serum.

S.T.S.

See Serological Tests for Syphilis

Sugar

See Glucose

Sulfhemoglobin

Sulfhemoglobin is not ordinarily found in the blood. It is produced when sulfides combine with the hemoglobin in the blood. It is usually associated with the intake of excessive amounts of acetanilid or phenacetin.

Food and Drink Restrictions. None.

Procedure for Collecting Specimen. Venous blood is withdrawn and 5 cc. placed in an oxalate bottle or tube.

Laboratory Procedure. The blood is examined spectroscopically for the absorption bands in the transmitted light beam.

Possible Interfering Materials and Conditions. None reported yet.

Normal Range. Normally there is no sulfhemoglobin in the blood.

Sulfobromophthalein

See Bromsulphalein Retention

Sulfonamide Level

In treating patients with sulfonamide drugs it is often helpful to know the concentration of the drug in the blood in order to decide whether to change dosage. This test measures the concentration of sulfonamides in the blood and may be adapted to measure their concentration in any body fluid.

Food and Drink Restrictions. None.

Procedure for Collecting Specimen. Venous blood is withdrawn and 5 cc. placed in an oxalate bottle or tube. Other acceptable anticoagulants are heparin and EDTA.

Laboratory Procedure. A protein-free sample of serum is mixed with a reagent which gives a red color. The intensity of the color is measured in a colorimeter.

Possible Interfering Materials and Conditions. The levels of sulfonamides may be falsely elevated if the patient has been taking acetophenetidin, sometimes also called phenacetin. This drug is incorporated into many mixtures for over-the-counter and prescription sale. Most of the salicylate mixtures listed in table 27 contain acetophenetidin.

Normal Range. Normally there are no sulfonamides in the blood. The therapeutic level sought varies not only with the specific drug used but also with the invading microorganism. Some bacteria are much more sensitive to sulfonamides than others. In general, levels of between 5 and 15 mg. per 100 cc. of serum are sought.

Thorn Test

See Chapter 7

Thymol Turbidity

This a test of liver function. Normally, when serum is mixed with a saturated solution of thymol, turbidity is seen. The turbidity is usually increased in liver conditions, such as hepatitis, where the liver cells are damaged. In biliary obstruction without damage to the liver cells the turbidity is usually normal.

Food and Drink Restrictions. The patient must avoid foods and beverages containing fat (including milk) for at least 12 hours before the blood sample is drawn. Water may be taken freely.

Procedure for Collecting Specimen. Venous blood is withdrawn and 5 cc. placed in a test tube and allowed to coagulate. The test is performed on the serum.

Laboratory Procedure. A sample of serum is added to a saturated solution of thymol. The degree of turbidity produced is measured colorimetrically or by comparison with a set of standards.

Possible Interfering Materials and Conditions. The thymol turbidity reading may be increased by lipemia. Therefore, the patient should avoid fatty foods for at least 12 hours before blood is drawn for the test. Unfortunately, the usual hospital diet is high in fats, so that fasting may be necessary.

Normal Range. Less than 5 units.

Thyroxine Iodine

This test for thyroid function has the advantage of not being interfered with by the radiographic contrast media that make some other tests virtually useless. Since so many persons have received radiographic contrast media (table 22), this test is likely to become much more widely used. It measures the iodine in serum thyroxine, one of the main thyroid hormones, and thus provides an indication of the amount of the hormone in the serum. A lower than normal level suggests hypothyroidism. A higher than normal level suggests hyperthyroidism.

Food and Drink Restrictions. None.

Procedure for Collecting Specimen. Venous blood is withdrawn and 6 cc. placed in a test tube and allowed to coagulate. The test is performed on the serum.

Laboratory Procedure. Several different procedures are available. One measures the ability of the thyroxine from the patient's serum to displace radioactive thyroxine from thyroxine-binding globulin. Gas chromatographic methods are being developed and improved.

Possible Interfering Materials and Conditions. Diphenylhydantoin (Dilantin) and related drugs may interfere with the test results, giving spuriously low values. Oral contraceptives may give high values, but these may be true values, caused by the pharmacologic action of the drug.

Normal Range. The normal range of serum thyroxine iodine depends on the method used. The method of Murphy and Pattee has a normal range of 3.0 to 6.4 mcg./100 ml.

T_4 Iodine

See Thyroxine Iodine

Total Cholesterol

See Cholesterol

Total Protein

See Albumin, Globulin, Total Protein, A/G Ratio

TPI

See Treponemal Immobilization Test

Transaminase

See Serum Transaminase, Serum Glutamic Oxaloacetic Transaminase (SGOT), and Glutamic Pyruvic Transaminase (SGPT).

TSH

See Thyrotropin

Unsaturated Iron-Binding Capacity

See Iron-Binding Capacity

Urea Clearance

See Urea Clearance, Chapter 5

Urea Nitrogen—Blood Urea Nitrogen (B.U.N.)

This is a test of kidney function. Ordinarily the kidney readily excretes urea, the end product of protein metabolism, so that the blood urea concentration is fairly low. However, in certain kidney disorders the ability to excrete urea may be impaired, so that the concentration of urea nitrogen in the blood increases. This test gives essentially the same information as the non-protein nitrogen (N.P.N.) test and is somewhat more accurate. There is no reason to do both tests and in most hospitals one or the other is performed. A rising blood urea nitrogen level may portend mental clouding, confusion and disorientation, and the patient may eventually go into coma. Therefore, when the laboratory report indicates a rising blood urea nitrogen content, the nurse should be prepared to deal with a patient who might become difficult to handle.

Food and Drink Restrictions. None.

Procedure for Collecting Specimen. Venous blood is withdrawn and 5 cc. placed in an oxalate bottle or tube. Other acceptable anticoagulants are heparin and EDTA.

Laboratory Procedure. The urea is converted to ammonia by the enzyme urease. The amount of ammonia is then measured by titration with acid.

Possible Interfering Materials and Conditions. Many substances may cause elevations in the blood urea nitrogen concentrations. In most cases the elevation is real, caused by a drug effect on the kidney, but this is transient, and the level returns to normal soon after the drug is discontinued. Therefore, an elevation in blood urea nitrogen in patients receiving such drugs may not indicate pre-existing kidney disease. The drugs, listed mainly by official (generic) name, include:

Acetohexamide	Indomethacin
Amphotericin B	Kanamycin
Antimony compounds	Lipomul
Arsenicals	Methicillin
Bacitracin	Methyldopa
Blood, whole	Methysergide
Capreomycin	Nalidixic acid
Cephaloridine, high doses	Neomycin
Chloral hydrate (see	Pargyline
table 19)	Polymyxin B
Chlorthalidone	Radiopaque contrast media
Colistimethate	(see table 22 B)
Doxapram	Salicylates (see table 27)
Ethacrynic acid	Streptokinase-
Furosemide	streptodornase
Gentamicin	Thiazides
Guanethidine	Triamterene
Guanochlor	Vancomycin

Normal Range. 9 to 20 mg. of urea *nitrogen* per 100 cc. of blood. The amount of actual urea, as distinct from urea nitrogen, ranges from 19 to 40 mg. per 100 cc. of blood, but this values is seldom mentioned clinically.

Uric Acid

The test is usually performed to diagnose gout but it may also give significant results in other conditions. Uric acid is the end product of purine metabolism and purines come mainly from cell nuclei. The blood uric acid concentration in gout is high. The reason for this is unknown. The uric acid concentration may also be elevated in conditions involving marked cellular destruction such as leukemia, pneumonia and toxemias of pregnancy. With severe kidney damage there may be an elevated uric acid level because of decreased excretion. However, this does not afford an accurate index of kidney function.

Food and Drink Restrictions. None.

Procedure for Collecting Specimen. Venous blood is withdrawn and 5 cc. placed in an oxalate bottle or tube. Other acceptable anticoagulants are heparin and EDTA.

Laboratory Procedure. A sample of serum is added to a reagent or mixture of reagents which produce a blue color with uric acid. The intensity of the color is measured and the concentration of uric acid calculated.

Possible Interfering Materials and Conditions. The uric acid levels may be elevated by several drugs and treatments. Listed by official (generic) name these include:

Ascorbic acid	Pyrazinamide
Blood transfusions	Salicylates (see table 27)
Chlorothiazide	Theophylline
Nitrogen mustards	Thiazides

The levels may be lowered by:

Coumarin anticoagulants   Piperazine

Normal Range. 2 to 6 mg. per 100 cc. of serum.

Van den Bergh Test

See Bilirubin, Partition

V.D.R.L.

See Serological Tests for Syphilis

Wassermann

See Serological Tests for Syphilis

White Cell Count

See Blood Counts, White Cell Count

White Cell Differential Count

See Blood Counts, White Cell Differential Count

Zinc Sulfate Turbidity

This is primarily a test of liver function. Zinc sulfate precipitates the gamma globulins (a division of the serum globulins) in the serum. Since the amount of gamma globulin in the serum is elevated when the liver cells are damaged, this test is useful in evaluating the presence of liver damage. In cases of agammaglobulinemia (lack of gamma globulin) or hypogammaglobulinemia (low levels of gamma globulin) the zinc sulfate turbidity test may give lower than normal readings, suggesting the need for more precise measurements of gamma globulin levels.

Food and Drink Restrictions. None.

Procedure for Collecting Specimen. Venous blood is withdrawn and 5 cc. placed in a test tube and allowed to coagulate. The test is performed on the serum.

Laboratory Procedure. A measured volume of serum is added to a measured volume of zinc sulfate in an appropriate buffer. The turbidity is measured with a photoelectric colorimeter.

Possible Interfering Materials and Conditions. None reported yet.

Normal Range. 2 to 12 units.

4

Tests Performed on Cerebrospinal Fluid (C.S.F.)

Cerebrospinal fluid, often called spinal fluid, fills the ventricles of the brain and the central canal of the spinal cord. It acts as a fluid buffer which can enlarge or diminish in volume, when necessary, to protect the brain and spinal cord from compression injury when slight changes occur in the volume of the space enclosed by the cranium and spinal column. It may also help prevent traumatic jarring of the brain. The cerebrospinal fluid may also play a role in supplying oxygen and nutrients to the brain and cord and removing waste.

Cerebrospinal fluid is produced from blood by the choroid plexus, a highly vascular structure in the brain ventricles. It differs from filtrate of blood in several respects, and the exact mechanism by which it is formed is not known. It is, however, in osmotic equilibrium with the blood.

From the brain ventricles where it is produced, the cerebrospinal fluid passes slowly down the spinal canal and is slowly reabsorbed into the blood. Approximately 100 cc. of cerebrospinal fluid is normally present and usually that amount is produced and reabsorbed daily.

Because of its intimate association with the brain and spinal cord, cerebrospinal fluid is a useful indicator of disease in those organs.

Usually, cerebrospinal fluid is obtained by lumbar puncture. In this procedure the physician withdraws fluid after passing a needle between two lumbar vertebrae into the spinal canal. Lumbar puncture is to be viewed as the equivalent of a surgical operation. The same sterile precautions are essential. In some institutions the patient must sign a permission form before lumbar puncture can be performed.

In a few cases the cerebrospinal fluid is obtained by puncture of the cisterna magna. This requires insertion of a needle between the base of the skull and the first cervical vertebra. It can be done safely by physicians specially trained in this technique.

After the needle has entered the spinal canal the physician usually performs several tests of the cerebrospinal fluid pressure. Only after these have been done are fluid samples withdrawn for laboratory examination. The fluid samples are not placed in a single container, but into a series of small test tubes, usually 3 or 4, depending on the tests ordered. The test tubes must be kept in the correct order, since the first tubes are more likely to contain minute amounts of blood from the puncture. Those tests which would be affected by small amounts of blood are therefore performed on fluid contained in the last tubes.

Cell Count

This test often indicates the presence of infection, such as meningitis. It is usually performed immediately following lumbar puncture and requires only about 15 minutes. The cell count is moderately increased (10 to 200 per cubic mm.) in such conditions as poliomyelitis, encephalitis and neurosyphilis. Cell counts of several thousand per cubic millimeter are found in most cases of meningitis.

Food and Drink Restrictions. None.

Procedure for Collecting Specimen. The physician places 1 to 2 cc. of cerebrospinal fluid in a special small test tube. Usually the third tube in the series is used, since it is less likely to contain minute amounts of blood.

Laboratory Procedure. The diluting fluid is drawn up to the first mark in the white cell pipette (used in white blood cell counts) and the spinal fluid is then drawn up to another mark. After mixing, a part of the mixture is placed in a counting chamber and the white cells counted with the aid of a microscope.

Possible Interfering Materials and Conditions. None reported yet.

Normal Range. 0 to 8 cells per cubic mm.

Chlorides

The cerebrospinal fluid chlorides are reduced in some types of meningitis, particularly tuberculous meningitis. Measurement of the chloride level may aid in differential diagnosis.

Food and Drink Restrictions. None.

Procedure for Collecting Specimen. The physician places 2 cc. of cerebrospinal fluid in a special small test tube.

Laboratory Procedure. The same as for blood chlorides.

Possible Interfering Materials and Conditions. None reported yet.

Normal Range. 720 to 760 mg. of sodium chloride per 100 cc. of spinal fluid. Note that this value is usually given in terms of mg. of sodium chloride per 100 cc., while the concentration of chlorides in serum is usually expressed as milliequivalents of chloride per liter.

If the value is expressed in terms of *chloride* alone, the normal range would be from about 435 to 465 mgm. per 100 cc., or about 123 to 132 milliequivalents per liter.

Colloidal Gold

This test is no longer in common use, since better methods of diagnosis are now available.

Culture

See Spinal Fluid Culture, Chapter 2

Protein

The spinal fluid protein is increased in several diseases of the central nervous system, especially meningitis and subarachnoid hemorrhage. Qualitative tests are now being replaced with simple quantitative tests of greater accuracy.

Food and Drink Restrictions. None.

Procedure for Collecting Specimen. The physician places 2 cc. of cerebrospinal fluid in a special small test tube. The last test tube of cerebrospinal fluid collected should be used for protein determination.

Laboratory Procedure. Several different procedures are available.

Possible Interfering Materials and Conditions. The spinal fluid protein level can appear falsely elevated by several drugs, if the measurement involves the use of the phospho-molybdic-phosphotungstic acid reagent (Folin-Ciocaltea reagent). The drugs which may have this effect are listed below (asterisk indicates official or common name):

*Acetophenetidin	*Phenacetin
*Aspirin	*Salicylates
*Chlorpromazine	(see table 27)
*Many drugs for mild	*Streptomycin
pain relief	*Sulfonamides
*Many headache remedies	Thorazine

If any local anesthetic gets into the spinal canal, this too will produce a spurious elevation of the cerebrospinal fluid protein when the Folin-Ciocalteau reagent is used.

Normal Range. 15 to 45 mg. per 100 cc. of spinal fluid.

Serological Tests

These tests are performed to discover the presence of neurosyphilis. A positive serological reaction of the spinal fluid almost always indicates neurosyphilis.

Food and Drink Restrictions. None.

Procedure for Collecting Specimen. The physician places 7 cc. of spinal fluid in a small test tube.

Laboratory Procedure. A Wassermann test is performed which is similar to that done on the blood.

Possible Interfering Materials and Conditions. None reported yet.

Normal Range. Normally the serological reaction is negative.

Sugar

Spinal fluid sugar is decreased in meningitis. This test is often useful in the differential diagnosis of central nervous system conditions.

Food and Drink Restrictions. None.

Procedure for Collecting Specimen. The physician places 2 cc. of cerebrospinal fluid in a special small test tube. If the test cannot be performed at once, breakdown of sugar must be prevented by preservation with a thymol crystal.

Laboratory Procedure. The degree to which the spinal fluid sample changes the color of cuprous oxide in the presence of molybdate-phosphate is compared to controls in a colorimeter.

Possible Interfering Materials and Conditions. None reported yet.

Normal Range. 50 to 80 mg. per 100 cc.

5

Tests Performed on Urine

Urine is formed by the kidneys. The glomeruli of the kidneys allow a filtrate of the blood plasma to pass into the tubules. The cells lining the tubules selectively reabsorb most of the filtrate. The tubule cells may also excrete certain substances into the urine being formed. During a 24-hour period a total of about 200 liters of fluid is filtered through the glomeruli and about 199 liters are reabsorbed by the tubules. The difference represents the urine excreted.

Although it is believed that the primary function of the kidneys is excretion of wastes, other functions are as important if not more so. They include regulation of ionic balance, acid-base balance and water balance of the body. Urine will vary widely in composition from time to time and such variations are indicative of good function and are not abnormal.

Some authorities divide tests of kidney function into three groups: those which test glomerular filtration (e.g., urea clearance), those which test tubular reabsorption (e.g., concentration and dilution tests), and those which test the excretion by the tubules (e.g., phenolsulfonphthalein excretion tests). Many kidney disorders, however, may involve both glomeruli and tubules, so that interpretation of the results of these tests requires considerable skill and experience. There are also many tests of urine which are done to evaluate the condition of organs other than the kidney.

Urine Preservatives. Urine specimens which cannot be sent directly to the laboratory should be protected against bacterial decomposition which can invalidate or confuse test results. This includes all 24-hour urine specimens. In general, refrigeration is an important method of preserving urine for short periods. In collecting 24 hour specimens, one should *not* leave the large urine bottle at the patient's bedside.

Instead, the large container should be kept in the refrigerator, and each voiding of urine during the 24 hour interval collected in fresh, clean smaller containers which are then poured promptly into the large refrigerated bottle. An alternative procedure is bringing the large refrigerated bottle to the patient for each voiding, and then replacing it in the refrigerator.

For some tests, it is also appropriate to use a chemical in order to reduce bacterial proliferation. In general, 10 ml. of toluene or 1 ml. of *glacial* acetic acid will preserve a liter of urine. However, for some tests, special preservatives are needed, since toluene or acetic acid would invalidate the results. The tests requiring special preservatives include:

Catecholamines: 10 cc. of concentrated hydrochloric acid are used for a 24-hour specimen.

17-ketosteroid excretion: 3 or more cc. of glacial acetic acid are needed for a 24-hour specimen.

Urobilinogen: 2 to 3 grams of sodium *carbonate* are used for each urine specimen.

Vanilmandelic Acid (VMA): 10 cc. of concentrated hydrochloric acid is used for a 24-hour specimen.

Aceto-Acetic Acid

See Diacetic Acid

Acetone

This test is important in the diagnosis of ketosis, a type of acidosis produced by faulty metabolism. In a condition such as diabetes, sugar is not utilized properly and excessive fat is metabolized. The fatty acids are broken down into aceto-acetic acid and B-hydroxybutyric acid. These cannot be completely disposed of by the tissues in the presence of impaired carbohydrate metabolism. They are converted to acetone which is then excreted by the kidneys. Acetone in the urine indicates a severe disorder of metabolism. The patient may exhibit symptoms of depression of the central nervous system.

Food and Drink Restrictions. None.

Procedure for Collecting Specimen. A urine sample is placed in a bottle and sent to the laboratory.

Laboratory Procedure. To the urine sample are added ammonium sulfate and a nitroprusside solution. Ammonia is then layered on top. A red to purple ring forms at the interface of the two layers if acetone is present.

Possible Interfering Materials and Conditions. If the patient has had a Bromsulphalein retention test (B.S.P.) or phenolsulfonphthalein test (P.S.P.) during the preceding 48 hours, there may be a false positive test for urine acetone.

The following may also give false positive tests for urine acetone (asterisk indicates official (generic) name):

DBI	*Levodopa
*L-dopa	*Metformin
Dopar	*Methionine
*Inositol	*Phenformin
*Larodopa	

Normal Range. Normally there is no acetone in the urine.

Addis Test

This is a method for determining the kind of kidney disease present. The number of cells and casts in the urine sediment are counted. A comparison of the amounts of each suggests the type of kidney disorder.

Food and Drink Restrictions. For 24 hours, 12 before and 12 during the test, all fluids, including water, coffee, milk, and soup are withheld. Otherwise, a normal diet may be taken.

Procedure for Collecting Specimen. If the patient is known to have severe renal disease with such signs as elevation of the urea nitrogen, this test should not be performed.

After approximately 12 hours without fluid, the patient urinates and the specimen is discarded. The time of voiding is noted. For the next 12 hours all urine specimens are voided directly into a large, clean, dry bottle and the total specimen collected. The bottle is kept sealed and in a cool place until the end of the test, when it is delivered to the laboratory.

Laboratory Procedure. The entire specimen is mixed thoroughly. Then a sample of urine is centrifuged and the sediment examined microscopically. The white blood cells, red blood cells and casts are counted, and the total number of each excreted in the 12-hour period is calculated.

Possible Interfering Materials and Conditions. None reported yet.

Normal Range:

> Per 12-hour specimen—
> Red blood cells   0 to 450,000
> White blood cells   30,000 to 1,000,000
> Hyaline casts   0 to 5,000

Albumin, Qualitative

Ordinarily the albumin in the blood does not pass through the glomerular wall into the urine. However, in several conditions such as kidney disease, hypertension, severe heart failure or drug toxicity, albumin appears in the urine. It may also be seen in orthostatic albuminuria which is not a disease. Therefore, the test is not specific but indicates that more precise tests are needed.

Food and Drink Restrictions. None.

Procedure for Collecting Specimen. A urine specimen is placed in a bottle and sent to the laboratory.

Laboratory Procedure. There are several procedures in use.

Possible Interfering Materials and Conditions. Many drugs are capable of producing a positive test for urine albumin. Some of these test results may be spurious, others may represent a small transient amount of kidney dysfunction. Because the number of drugs having this effect is so large, it is impractical to try to include the brand names;

therefore, only the official or the common names are listed here:

Aminophylline
Aminosalicylic acid
Amphotericin B
Antimony compounds
Arsenicals
Bacitracin
Bismuth triglycollamate
Capreomycin
Carbarsone
Carbutamide
Carinamide
Chlorpropamide
Colistimethate
Diatrizoate (may produce 4 + levels)
Dihydrotachysterol
Dithiazanine
Doxapram
Edathamil
Ethosuximide
Gentamycin
Gold salts
Griseofulvin
Iodoalphionic acid
Iodopanoic acid
Isoniazid
Kanamycin
Mefenamic acid

Metahexamide
Metaxalone
Methenamine, large doses
Methicillin
Methsuximide
Neomycin
Paraldehyde
Paramethadione
Para-aminosalicylic acid
Penicillamine
Penicillin (large doses)
Phenacemide
Phenindione
Polymyxin B
Pyrazolone derivatives
Radiographic contrast media (may produce 4 + levels)
Salicylates (see table 27)
Sulfisoxazole
Sulfones
Suramin
Thiosemicarbazones
Tolbutamide
Trimethadione
Viomycin
Vitamin D

Normal Range. In 5 to 15 per cent of normal individuals small amounts of albumin are sometimes found in the urine with no disease present. This has been termed orthostatic or postural albuminuria.

Albumin, Quantitative

This test is performed to discover the amount of albumin lost daily in the urine. This information may be helpful in attempting to restore protein balance.

Food and Drink Restrictions. None.

Procedure for Collecting Specimen. The urine excreted during a 24-hour period is collected in a clean bottle and sent to the laboratory.

Laboratory Procedure. Several methods may be used. They involve the addition of reagents which precipitate the albumin. The amount of precipitate or degree of turbidity is then compared to standards.

Possible Interfering Materials and Conditions. Many drugs are capable of producing a positive test for urine albumin. Some of these test results may be spurious, others may represent a small transient amount of kidney dysfunction. Because the number of drugs having this effect is so large, it is impractical to try to include the brand names, therefore only the official (or common) names are listed here:

Aminophylline
Aminosalicylic acid
Amphotericin B
Antimony compounds
Arsenicals
Bacitracin
Bismuth triglycollamate
Capreomycin
Carbarsone
Carbutamide
Carinamide
Chlorpropamide
Colistimethate
Diatrizoate (may produce 4+ levels)
Dihydrotachysterol
Dithiazanine
Doxapram
Edathamil
Ethosuximide
Gentamycin
Gold salts
Griseofulvin
Iodoalphionic acid
Iodopanoic acid
Isoniazid
Kanamycin
Mefenamic acid
Metahexamide
Metaxalone
Methenamine, large doses
Methicillin
Methsuximide
Neomycin

Paraldehyde
Paramethadione
Para-aminosalicylic acid
Penicillamine
Penicillin (large doses)
Phenacemide
Phenindione
Polymyxin B
Pyrazolone derivatives
Radiographic contrast me-
dia (may produce 4+ levels)
Salicylates (see table 27)
Sulfisoxazole
Sulfones
Suramin
Thiosemicarbazones
Tolbutamide
Trimethadione
Viomycin
Vitamin D

Normal Range. In 5 to 15 per cent of normal individuals small amounts of albumin are sometimes found in the urine with no disease present. This has been termed orthostatic or postural albuminuria.

Amino Acids

This series of tests for the excess of particular amino acids in the urine is used to determine whether one or another type of condition, often congenital in nature, may be present. Two main types of conditions lead to excess amino acids in the urine. The so-called "renal type" results from a defect in the renal tubules. In some defects, for example, the Fanconi syndrome, all amino acids are excreted in the urine in increased amounts. In other renal tubular defects, there may be an increased excretion of all or some amino acids, but a much greater excretion of one or more particular amino acids. When the aminoaciduria is caused by a defect in the renal tubule, the plasma levels of the amino acids are generally normal.

The second type of aminoaciduria is called the "overflow" type. In this condition, abnormal metabolism of one or more amino acids leads to an extremely high level in the plasma, so that normal tubular reabsoption cannot handle the load, and some spills over into the urine. Many of these overflow aminoacidurias are caused by congenital metabolic defects. Phenylketonuria is perhaps the best-known example.

Chromatography and electrophoresis are employed whenever aminoaciduria is suspected, and the results of the test generally indicate the kinds of amino acids being excreted in excess. They do not, however, distinguish between renal and overflow types. To make that distinction, studies of the plasma are also needed.

In some cases, additional tests are applicable to specific types of aminoaciduria.

Many diverse conditions can cause aminoaciduria, including congenital disorders, heavy metal and other types of poisoning, severe burns, and liver and kidney diseases. The major causes of aminoaciduria are summarized in table 1.

Food and Drink Restrictions. None reported.

Procedure for Collecting Specimen. Usually a fresh urine specimen is needed, although in some hospitals, a 24-hour specimen may be required. This test is frequently performed on infants, and particular care must be exercised to prevent any contamination of the urine by feces.

Laboratory Procedure. The amino acids are identified in the urine by high-voltage paper electrophoresis and paper chromatography.

Possible Interfering Materials and Conditions. The screening test for homogentisic acid (P.156) may produce a false positive result if the patient has received salicylates (table 27) in the preceding 3 days. However, the chromatographic test should give accurate results.

The screening test for phenylketonuria (P.168) may be interfered with if the patient has received phenothiazines (table 25), or salicylates (table 27). However, the chromatographic test should give accurate results.

If protein hydrolysate is given intravenously, there will be a generalized aminoaciduria.

Normal Range. A normal adult excretes from 300 to 650 mgm. of amino acids in the urine every 24 hours. This contains from 50 to 200 mgm. of amino acid nitrogen. The relative concentrations of the different amino acids vary somewhat, and are seldom measured directly. Abnormalities are detected by comparing the test chromatogram with a normal pattern.

TABLE 1

MAIN TYPES OF AMINOACIDURIA

Disease	Type of Disease	Mechanism of Aminoaciduria	Amino Acids in Excess in Urine
alkaptonuria	congenital	overflow	homogentisic acid
aminoaciduria of liver disease	acquired	overflow	all
argininosuccinic aciduria	congenital	overflow	argininosuccinic acid, citrulline
burns, severe	acquired	renal	several
citrullinemia	congenital	overflow	citrulline
cystathioninuria	congenital	overflow	cystathionine
cystinuria	congenital	renal	cystine, lysine, arginine, ornithine
Fanconi syndrome	acquired	renal	several
fructuose intolerance	congenital	renal	several
galactosemia	congenital	renal	all
glycinuria	congenital	renal	glycine
Hartnup disease	congenital	renal	most
heavy metal poisoning	acquired	renal	several
histidinemia	congenital	overflow	histidine
homocystinuria	congenital	overflow	methionine, hemocystine
hydroxyprolinemia	congenital	overflow	hydroxyproline
hyperglycinemia	congenital	overflow	glycine, and sometimes leucine
hyperlysinemia	congenital	overflow	lysine
hyperprolinemia	congenital	overflow	proline
hypervalinemia	congenital	overflow	valine
hypophosphatasia	congenital	overflow	phosphoethanolamine
maleic acid poisoning	acquired	renal	several
maple-syrup urine disease	congenital	overflow	valine, leucine and isoleucine
Oasthouse urine disease	congenital	overflow	phenylalanine, methionine, valine, leucine, isoleucine, and tyrosine

Disease	Type of Disease	Mechanism of Aminoaciduria	Amino Acids in Excess in Urine
oxalic acid poisoning	acquired	renal	several
phenol poisoning	acquired	renal	several
phenylketonuria	congenital	overflow	phenylalanine
rickets	acquired	renal	several
scurvy	acquired	renal	several
starvation	acquired	overflow	beta-amino-isobutyric acid
tyrosinosis	congenital	overflow	tyrosine
von Gierke's disease	congenital	renal	several
Wilson's disease	congenital	renal	all

Amylase (See Amylase, Chapter 3)

This is a test for pancreatic diseases in which the digestive enzymes of the pancreas may escape into the surrounding tissue, producing necrosis with severe pain and inflammation. These enzymes, including amylase, are found in the serum, where they can be measured (see P.37), and are excreted in the urine. The serum amylase levels tend to remain high for a short time, sometimes only a few hours, while the urine levels remain high for about a week. Therefore, when the physician suspects that the time for finding the elevated serum amylase level might have passed, he may order a urinary amylase determination.

Food and Drink Restrictions. None.

Procedure for Collecting Specimen. A timed collection is required. Institutions vary as to the time intervals used. Some use a 2-hour specimen, others a 12- or 24-hour specimen. It is essential that the exact times of the beginning and the end of the collection period be recorded and sent to the laboratory with the specimen. The *beginning* of a collection period is the time when a patient empties his bladder, with that specimen being discarded. All subsequent urine specimens are saved, including the one at the end of the collection period.

It is not clear which, if any, preservatives are suitable for these urine specimens, and which might interfere with the test. Unless the laboratory specifies that a preservative may be used, it would be best to avoid the preservative and keep the urine sample refrigerated until it is sent to the laboratory.

Laboratory Procedure. Starch in solution is hydrolysed by the urinary amylase. A control solution in which the hydrolysis of the starch is prevented is allowed to react with iodine, producing a blue color. The extent to which the urinary amylase prevents the blue color from appearing in the test sample as compared to the control is the measure of urinary amylase level.

Possible Interfering Materials and Conditions. The data on possible interfering materials and conditions for urinary amylase measurements and interpretations is incomplete and unclear. It seems prudent to assume that those materials and conditions that interfere with *serum* amylase level interpretations may likewise interfere with urinary level interpretations.

The following drugs, therefore, might produce elevations of urinary amylase levels (asterisk indicates official (generic) name):

* Bethanechol
* Codeine
  Demerol
* Ethyl alcohol (large amounts)
* Meperidine
* Methyl alcohol (large amounts)
* Morphine
  Myocholine (bethanechol)
* Narcotic drugs
  Urecholine (bethanechol)

There may be a spurious decrease in apparent urinary amylase levels if the urine specimens become contaminated with fluorides.

The following conditions may produce elevated urinary amylase levels:

Mumps
Diseases of salivary glands and ducts
Some intestinal obstructions

Any contamination of the urinary specimen by saliva may result in a spuriously high urinary amylase level. Such contamination might come from improper pipetting, or from spitting, coughing, sneezing, or even talking near the uncovered specimen.

Normal Range. The normal range is under 270 units *per hour.*

Aschheim-Zondek Test

This is a test for pregnancy. During pregnancy hormones are produced and excreted in the urine. When the urine of a pregnant woman is injected into immature animals, these hormones can stimulate the animal's ovaries, so that they simulate early pregnancy in the animal. A quantitative Aschheim-Zondek test is sometimes performed to diagnose teratoma and chorionepithelioma (malignant tumors).

Food and Drink Restrictions. None.

Procedure for Collecting Specimen. About 75 cc. of morning urine is placed in a bottle and sent to the laboratory.

Laboratory Procedure. Small amounts of urine are injected into immature female mice daily for 3 days. On the fifth day the animals are killed and the ovaries examined. If there are hemorrhagic follicles, the test is positive.

Possible Interfering Materials and Conditions. In teratoma and chorionepithelioma (malignant tumors), there may be a positive Aschheim-Zondek test. Interference with the test by drugs has not yet been reported. Apparently those drugs that interfere with the frog tests do not interfere with tests using mammals.

Normal Range. In the absence of pregnancy this test is negative.

Ascorbic Acid (Vitamin C) Tolerance (Urine)

See Ascorbic Acid Tolerance (Blood)

This test measures the degree of ascorbic acid deficiency. Although not as widely performed as it once was it can provide important clinical information. We recognize now that some persons with seemingly adequate diets, and even some receiving supplemental vitamins, may have a partial deficiency in ascorbic acid. This may occur in patients with severe burns, infection, or malignacy. A partial deficiency of ascorbic acid can interfere with wound healing, body defenses, and recovery.

In normal persons, when a large dose of ascorbic acid is given intravenously, about 30% or more will be excreted in the urine. In cases of relative ascorbic acid deficiency, much less will be excreted.

Food and Drink Restrictions. For 24 hours before the test, the patient must avoid foods high in ascorbic acid. Water may be taken as desired.

Procedure for Collecting Specimen. In recent years, the procedure has been simplified so that a 5- or 6-hour urine specimen is now used instead of a 24-hour specimen. The patient empties his bladder, and this specimen is discarded. All subsequent specimens are collected in a bottle containing glacial acetic acid, 1 cc. of acid to 9 cc. of urine.

The patient receives the ascorbic acid orally or intravenously. In the oral method, 11 mg. per kg. of body weight is dissolved in a glass of water and swallowed. All urine voided during the next 6 hours (5 in some hospitals) is collected in the bottle with acetic acid and sent immediately to the laboratory at the end of the period.

In the intravenous method, the physician injects the test dose mixed in an appropriate solution. There are variations in the doses used from 500 mg. to 1 Gm. All urine specimens during the next 5 hours are collected and sent immediately to the laboratory at the end of the period.

This test may be done in conjunction with the blood test (P.40).

Laboratory Procedure. The amount of ascorbic acid in the urine is measured photometrically after chemical modification.

Possible Interfering Materials and Conditions. None reported yet.

Normal Range. For the oral test — excretion of 10% of the administered amount.

For the intravenous test — excretion of 30 to 40% of the administered amount.

Bacterial Count

The primary use of bacterial count of the urine is to distinguish between true infection of the urinary tract and contamination of specimens by bacteria residing near the urethral opening. In the past, catheterization was used to get urine specimens that were supposedly free of contamination. However, the disclosure that catheterization has a substantial risk (around 5%) of producing a urinary tract infection where none existed before has made it prudent to avoid catheterization. The techniques used to obtain urine specimens for culture may permit skin bacteria to contaminate the culture, but a count of the bacteria can usually reveal whether they came from an infection or from the skin. Urine bacteria counts of over 100,000 per ml. of urine generally mean that there is a significant urinary tract infection. Counts of less than 10,000 bacteria generally signify contamination of the sample, without true infection of the urinary tract. Counts between 10,000 and 100,000 per ml. of urine are inconclusive, and should be repeated.

In some circumstances, bacterial counts might be used to follow the course of a patient being treated for a known urinary tract infection.

Food and Drink Restrictions. None.

Procedure for Collecting Specimen. One of the crucial aspects of this test is the need to minimize any delay between the collection of the specimen and the delivery to the laboratory.

To collect a specimen from a male patient, the patient starts to urinate, and then a mid-stream sample of urine is caught in a sterile container.

To collect a specimen from a female patient, the entire vulvar area is first cleansed carefully, using a dilute solution of benzalkonium (Zephiran) or hexachloraphene. Both should not be used on the same patient, however. Then, the cleansed area is rinsed with sterile water, being careful not to allow the water to flow from uncleansed to cleansed areas. Drying should be done by gentle patting with a sterile towel. Next, the labia are held apart, and after some urine has been passed, a sterile bottle is placed in the stream to catch a specimen. Specimens must then be taken to the laboratory at once.

Laboratory Procedure. A measured sample of the urine is plated out on culture media, and the number of bacterial colonies growing on a predetermined area of the media is counted. Since each colony arises from a single bacterium, it is possible to calculate the number of bacteria in a ml. of urine.

Possible Interfering Materials and Conditions. Any antibiotic or chemotherapeutic agents taken by the patient may interfere with the count. If the benzalkonium or hexachloraphene is not rinsed off thoroughly, and contaminates the urine sample, spuriously low readings may be obtained.

Normal Range. Any counts under 10,000 per ml. of urine may be considered normal, and as resulting from external contamination.

Bence Jones Protein

This is a test for certain tumors. Bence Jones protein is an unusual type of protein molecule with a molecular weight of about 35,000 as compared to 70,000 for albumin. It coagulates on heating at about 45° C. and redissolves at about 100° C. It is excreted in large amounts in the urine in most cases of multiple myeloma. It may also be found in other types of bone tumors.

Food and Drink Restrictions. None.

Procedure for Collecting Specimen. A urine sample is placed in a bottle and sent to the laboratory.

Laboratory Procedure. The urine sample is acidified to pH 5 and heated to 45° to 70° C If coagulation of protein is seen, the urine is heated to 100° C If the coagulum is due to Bence Jones protein, it redissolves at 100° C and recoagulates at 70° C or less.

Possible Interfering Materials and Conditions. Bence Jones protein may appear in the urine of patients who have taken out-dated tetracycline.

In Waldenströms macroglobulinemia, Bence Jones protein may also appear in the urine.

Normal Range. Normally, small amounts of Bence Jones protein may be found in the urine using highly sensitive techniques, but the amount is too small to be observed with usual techniques in the absence of disease.

Bile and Bilirubin

This is a test of liver function. Bile pigments and acids are found in the urine when there is obstruction of the biliary tract. Bilirubin (the main pigment) is found alone when there is excessive hemolysis of the red blood cells.

Food and Drink Restrictions. None.

Procedure for Collecting Specimen. A urine specimen is placed in a bottle and sent to the laboratory. The test for bile acids cannot be performed if the urine specimen has been preserved with thymol.

Laboratory Procedure. Several tests are available. One of the most widely used employs prepackaged test tablets.

Possible Interfering Materials and Conditions. There may be a false positive test for bile if the patient has taken chlorzoxazone (Paraflex).

There may be an elevation of urine bilirubin if the patient has received certain drugs. The elevation may be due to transient interference with liver function, and does not indicate permanent liver disease. These drugs, listed by official (generic) names, include:

Acetophenazine   Phenazopyridine
Chlorprothixene   Phenothiazines, some
Ethoxazene

Normal Range. Normally bile acids and bilirubin are not found in the urine.

Blood

Blood in the urine may appear as intact red blood cells (hematuria) or dissolved hemoglobin derived from destroyed red blood cells (hemoglobinuria). Hematuria comes from bleeding somewhere along the urinary tract from glomerulus to urethra. The site of bleeding and its cause are determined by more precise testing methods. Hemoglobinuria usually arises from conditions outside the urinary tract. The red cells are hemolyzed and the dissolved hemoglobin in the plasma is excreted by the kidney. It is seen in severe burns, transfusion reactions, severe malaria (blackwater fever), poisoning, and paroxysmal hemoglobinuria.

Food and Drink Restrictions. None.

Procedure for Collecting Specimen. A urine specimen is placed in a bottle and sent to the laboratory.

Laboratory Procedure. Intact red blood cells are identified by centrifuging the urine and examining the sediment microscopically.

Hemoglobin is now identified by special paper strips impregnated with orthotolidine. Few laboratories use the older methods.

Possible Interfering Materials and Conditions. A positive test may result from myoglobin in the urine, or from large amounts of bacteria or of pus in the urine.

A false negative test can result when a patient receives large amounts of ascorbic acid, either as therapeutic vitamin supplements, or parenteral tetracyclines in which ascorbic acid is used as a preservative.

A large number of drugs may cause enough urinary bleeding to produce a positive test for blood in the urine.

Although this is a true result, it can be misleading if the causative role of the drug is not understood. This bleeding does not indicate any basic urinary tract disease, and does not warrant extensive diagnostic studies. When the drug is withdrawn, the bleeding soon stops. Drugs that may cause such bleeding, listed by official (generic) name, include:

Aminosalicyclic acid
Amphotericin B
Bacitracin
Chloroguanide
Colchicine
Corticosteroids
Coumarin anticoagulants
Cyclophosphamide
Gold salts
Indomethacin
Kanamycin
Mandelic acid derivatives
Mefenamic acid
Mephenesin
Mersalyl theophylline
Methenamine
Oxyphenbutazone
Methicillin
Para-aminosalicylic acid
Phenindione derivatives
Phenylbutazone
Phytonadione
Polymyxin B
Probenecid
Proguanil
Pyrazolone derivatives
Sulfonamides
Sulfones
Suramin
Thiazides
Viomycin

Normal Range. Normally, a few red blood cells may be seen per high power field. In the female, blood due to menstrual flow may be found. A catheterized specimen may contain blood because of urethral bleeding from the trauma of inserting the catheter.

Calcium Test (Sulkowitch)

This test measures roughly the amount of calcium in the urine. In hypoparathyroidism the urinary excretion of calcium is decreased. This test is therefore useful in cases of tetany to determine quickly whether the cause is hypoparathyroidism.

Food and Drink Restrictions. None.

Procedure for Collecting Specimen. A urine sample is placed in a bottle and sent to the laboratory.

Laboratory Procedure. To a sample of urine is added an equal volume of Sulkowitch reagent. The extent of precipitation indicates roughly the amount of calcium. Absence of a precipitate indicates an abnormally low serum calcium.

Possible Interfering Materials and Conditions. The urine calcium levels may be spuriously elevated if the patient has received any of the following:

Cholestyramine resin   Parathyroid injection
Dihydrotachysterol   Vitamin D
Nandrolone

There may be interference with the test if the patient has received:

Thiazides   Viomycin

Normal Range. A fine white precipitate indicates a normal concentration of serum calcium.

Catecholamines

This is a test for the presence of pheochromocytoma, a rare tumor of the chromaffin cells of the adrenal medulla and other parts of the sympathetic nervous system. Catecholamines are substances with chemical structures similar to those of epinephrine (Adrenalin) and norepinephrine (arterenol). When produced in the body, some of the unchanged material and some of the breakdown products containing the basic catecholamine structure are excreted in the urine. In cases of pheochromocytoma, the urinary levels of catecholamines are usually 3 to 100 times greater than normal. A correct diagnosis is usually life-saving, since pheochromocytomas produce severe hypertension, which is cured when the pheochromocytoma is removed surgically. In some psychiatric patients, catecholamine levels in the urine are slightly higher than normal, but not enough to be confused with pheochromocytoma. On the other hand, in the future, the slight catecholamine level elevations in psychiatric disorders may prove of considerable clinical and research value.

Food and Drink Restrictions. None.

Procedure for Collecting Specimen. The patient should take no drugs for 3 days before the beginning of the test. Notify the laboratory that the test has been ordered. Place 10 cc. of *concentrated* hydrochloric acid in a large bottle for a 24-hour urine specimen. Observe precautions to avoid spattering any of the acid on persons or materials. If possible, obtain a prepared bottle from the laboratory. Make sure there is no acid on the outside. Cap the bottle and place in the refrigerator. Collect in ordinary clean urine bottles each urine specimen voided by the patient in a 24-hour period. As soon as each specimen is voided, pour it carefully into the large refrigerated bottle, and replace the latter in the refrigerator.

Laboratory Procedure. The procedure for measuring catecholamines is so complicated that relatively few hospitals perform it themselves. Instead, they send the samples to specialized laboratories. This means that results are delayed. The basic method used is column chromatography, oxidation, and then photofluorometry.

Possible Interfering Materials and Conditions. The urine catecholamine levels may be spuriously elevated by bananas and coffee, and also by many drugs. These drugs, listed by generic (official) name, include:

Demethylchlortetracycline
Epinephrine by inhalation
Hydralazine
Methenamine
Methyldopa
Nicotinic acid, large doses
Quinidine
Quinine
Riboflavin, large doses
Salicylates (see table 27)
Tetracyclines
Vitamin B complex, large doses

Severe anxiety or anger may produce elevations of catecholamine levels.

Normal Range. Normally, the urinary excretion of catecholamines is less than 140 micrograms in 24 hours.

Chlorides, Quantitative

This examination is performed to evaluate the urinary excretion of chlorides. It is useful in the management of cardiac patients on low salt diets and in adjusting fluid and ion balance in postoperative cases.

Food and Drink Restrictions. None.

Procedure for Collecting Specimen. The total urine excreted over a 24-hour period is collected in a large bottle.

Laboratory Procedure. A simplified test, using a manufactured tablet, is now replacing the more complex analytical chemical techniques.

Possible Interfering Materials and Conditions. There may be a spurious elevation of urine chloride levels if the patient has taken bromides.

Normal Range. This may vary considerably with salt intake and with perspiration. In general, most of the ingested chloride, less that lost in perspiration, is excreted in the urine. Thus there is really no "normal" or "abnormal" range and the values obtained in this test are significant only in relation to the balance between intake and output. Usually there are about 9 Gm. of sodium chloride per liter of urine.

Concentration and Dilution

These tests measure the ability of the kidneys to concentrate and dilute urine, an indication of their functional capacity. Inadequate concentration or dilution of urine indicates some disorder of the tubules of the kidneys.

Procedure for Collecting Specimen. The procedures vary in different institutions. A fairly common one is the following:

First night

1. At supper the patient is restricted to 1 glass of fluid.

2. Thereafter no food or drink is given until the end of the test.

3. The patient remains in bed as much as possible.

4. Before going to sleep the patient empties the bladder and the urine is discarded.

5. On arising the patient passes a urine specimen which is saved.

6. Second and third specimens are collected 1 and 2 hours later. The exact time of voiding each specimen is recorded.

7. After the third specimen the patient may have food and drink.

Second night

8. A regular supper is eaten.

9. No food or drink allowed thereafter, except as specified.

10. The patient is kept in bed as much as possible.

11. On awakening in the morning, the patient empties the bladder and the urine specimen is discarded.

12. After urination the patient is given 5 glasses of fluid to drink within 45 minutes. The fluid may be water, lemonade or weak tea.

13. Urine is collected 1, 2, 3 and 4 hours after the patient has started drinking.

14. After the 4-hour specimen has been collected, the patient may have food and drink.

Laboratory Procedure. The specific gravity of each urine specimen is measured with a urinometer.

Possible Interfering Materials and Conditions. None reported yet.

Normal Range. For concentration phase, specific gravity of 1.026 or over. For dilution phase, specific gravity of about 1.003 in first urine specimen, gradually increasing thereafter.

Corticosteroids

See 17 Hydroxy Corticosteroids

Creatinine Clearance

This is a test of kidney glomerular function. When the serum creatinine level is in the normal range, 0.6 to 1.3 mg. per 100 cc., the urinary excretion of creatinine depends almost entirely on the glomeruli. However, if serum creatinine levels rise above normal, the tubules excrete significant amounts of it, so that interpretation of creatinine clearance becomes complex. The creatinine clearance test is useful in two basic situations. It can be an early sign of glomerular damage, producing abnormal results when the serum creatinine levels are still within normal limits. Also, it can be used to follow the course of known glomerular disease and to evaluate the effects of treatment.

Food and Drink Restrictions. Beginning at least 6 hours before the test, and continuing throughout the test, the patient should not receive any meat, poultry, fish, tea, or coffee. Otherwise, he may have ordinary hospital foods. His water intake should be at least 100 cc. per hour for the test period.

Procedure for Collecting Specimen. 1. Urine — On the morning of the test, the patient empties his bladder completely, and the exact time is noted. This urine sample is discarded. The patient drinks a glass of water, and continues to drink water at a rate of at least 100 cc. per hour. ALL urine passed during the next 24 hours is collected without any preservative, but is stored in a refrigerator. The exact time of the last voiding is also noted. Some hospitals use a collection period of less than 24 hours.

2. Blood — On the morning of the test, venous blood is withdrawn and 6 cc. placed in a test tube and allowed to coagulate.

Laboratory Procedure. The serum creatinine level is measured as described under creatinine, as well as the amount of creatinine in the 24-hour urine specimen. From these measurements, the volume of serum cleared of creatinine per minute is calculated.

Possible Interfering Materials and Conditions. Foods with high creatinine content (meat, poultry, fish) may interfere with the results. Coffee and tea may interfere because of their diuretic effects. Strenuous excercise may also interfere. Diuretic drugs may give spurious results, and should not be given for at least a day before the test and during the test.

Normal Range. The normal creatinine clearance is 100 to 140 ml. per minute.

Culture

See Urine Culture, Chapter 2

Diacetic (Aceto-Acetic) Acid

This test is used in the diagnosis of metabolic ketosis. Like acetone, diacetic acid is produced when glucose is not properly utilized, and excessive fat is metabolized. A positive test for diacetic acid indicates a more severe degree of ketosis (acidosis) than a positive acetone test alone. The patient may develop weakness, headache, thirst, air hunger, epigastric pain and vomiting. These symptoms may progress to restlessness and confusion or to symptoms of central nervous system depression. If untreated, coma and death may ensue.

Food and Drink Restrictions. None.

Procedure for Collecting Specimen. A urine sample is placed in a bottle and sent to the laboratory.

Laboratory Procedure. To a sample of urine in a test tube is added a 10% solution of ferric chloride. A purple color indicates diacetic acid.

Possible Interfering Materials and Conditions. A false positive test for diacetic acid may result from one of the following:

L-dopa
Drugs derived from coal tar
Phenothiazines (see table 25)
Salicylates (see table 27)

Normal Range. Normally there is no diacetic acid in the urine.

d-Xylose Tolerance Test (oral)

See Xylose

Fermentation Test for Sugar

This test differentiates between the various kinds of sugar in the urine. Not all sugar found in the urine is glucose. Other sugars which may be present are fructose, galactose, lactose, and various pentoses (sugars with 5 carbons). The presence of these sugars does not indicate diabetes, but usually means there is some other metabolic defect. It may be important in some cases to make sure whether or not the sugar found in the urine is glucose.

Food and Drink Restrictions. None.

Procedure for Collecting Specimen. A urine sample is placed in a bottle and sent to the laboratory.

Laboratory Procedure. The urine sample, to which yeast is added, is placed in a special fermentation tube and kept in an incubator for a period of time. If glucose is present, carbon dioxide will be produced through fermentation and will be readily visible because of the shape of the container.

Possible Interfering Materials and Conditions. None reported yet.

Normal Range. Normally there is no sugar in the urine.

Friedman Test

This is a test for pregnancy and is basically the same as the Aschheim-Zondek, but employs a female rabbit.

Frog Test for Pregnancy

This test is based on the observation that the hormones excreted in the urine during pregnancy, if injected into a male frog will usually cause it to discharge spermatozoa within 2 to 4 hours. This test is rapid and economical, and is therefore widely performed. It has two disadvantages. During the early spring, the frogs have spermatozoa in their urine normally, so that other tests may have to be substituted. In addition, it has been noted that the urine of patients receiving drugs of the phenothiazine group (tranquilizers) often give false positive results. Like other pregnancy tests, this one can be positive in the presence of teratomas and chorionepitheliomas (malignant tumors).

Food and Drink Restrictions. None.

Procedure for Collecting Specimen. A urine specimen is placed in a bottle and sent to the laboratory. Morning urine is preferable.

Laboratory Procedure. A small amount of urine is injected into a male frog. After several hours, some of the frog's cloacal contents are examined under the microscope for spermatozoa. Their presence is a positive result.

Possible Interfering Materials and Conditions. Teratomas and chorionepitheliomas (malignancies) can produce positive results.

A false positive test may result if the patient has received any of the following drugs in the preceding two months (asterisk indicates official or common name):

*Chlorpromazine	Sparine
*Promazine	Thoradex
Prozine	Thorazine

It is not yet clear whether related drugs also produce false positive results.

Normal Range. In the absence of pregnancy, this test is normally negative.

Glucose

See Sugar

Glucose Tolerance

See Glucose Tolerance, Chapter 3

Gravindex

See Immunologic Test for Pregnancy.

Heroin

See Morphine

5-HIAA

See 5-Hydroxyindoleacetic Acid

Hogben

This is another test for pregnancy, in which a female South African toad is the test animal. The advantage of this test over the Aschheim-Zondek and Friedman tests it that the animal does not have to be killed and can be used repeatedly. Like the other pregnancy tests, this one can also be positive in the presence of teratoma and chorionepithelioma.

Food and Drink Restrictions. None.

Procedure for Collecting the Specimen. A sample of morning urine is placed in a bottle and sent to the laboratory.

Laboratory Procedure. A small amount of the urine is injected into a female toad. If the toad releases eggs within 24 hours, the test is considered positive.

Possible Interfering Materials and Conditions. Teratoma and chorionepithelioma (malignancies) can produce positive test results. A false positive test may result if the patient has received any of the following drugs in the preceding two months. (asterisk indicates official or common name):

°Chlorpromazine	Sparine
°Promazine	Thoradex
Prozine	Thorazine

It is not yet clear whether related drugs also produce false positive results.

Normal Range. In the absence of pregnancy, this test is usually negative.

Homogentisic Acid

This is a test for alkaptonuria, a rather rare metabolic disease. In this condition, the oxidation of tyrosine does not proceed fully along the normal pathways, and an intermediary metabolite, homogentisic acid, is excreted in the urine. The urine is normally colored when voided, but turns dark on standing. Furthermore, pigment is deposited in the eye, ear and nose and tendons of the hand. One or more of these signs may bring the patient to medical attention. Alkaptonuria is not a particularly dangerous condition. Its major disadvantage is the development of arthritis in later life. There is no specific treatment available at this time. An accurate diagnosis of alkaptonuria is of great benefit to the patient and his family, however, since it should relieve any concern that a fatal or life-shortening disorder may be present.

Food and Drink Restrictions. None.

Procedure for Collecting Specimen. Ordinarily, any fresh urine sample is sufficient for this test.

Laboratory Procedure. Several procedures are available. The simplest is the addition of alkali, which turns the urine black. Homogentisic acid will also give a positive reaction to the Benedict reagent in a common test for sugar.

Possible Interfering Materials and Conditions. The level of homogentisic acid may seem falsely elevated if the patient has received salicylates (table 27) in the preceding three days.

Normal Range. Normally there is no homogentisic acid in the urine. Salicylates may produce milligram quantities of gentisic acid, a similar material. However, in alkaptonuria, much larger amounts of homogentisic acid are found.

5-Hydroxyindoleacetic Acid (5-HIAA)

This is a test for the presence of a carcinoid tumor. These rare tumors are found mainly in the appendix, but occasionally in the small or large intestine. The cells of the carcinoid tumor secrete serotonin which is broken down to 5-hydroxy-indoleacetic acid, producing a marked elevation in the usual urinary levels of this material. Carcinoid tumors have a low degree of malignancy, so that reasonably prompt removal gives a high chance of complete cure. Recently, it was found that in a few rare cases, non-carcinoid tumors may also produce high urinary levels of 5-HIAA.

Food and Drink Restrictions. The patient must not eat any bananas for at least 3 days before the test.

Procedure for Collecting Specimen. The patient must be kept off most drugs for at least 3 full days before starting the collection of urine. The total urine for a 24-hour period is collected and sent to the laboratory. The specimen should be kept refrigerated.

Laboratory Procedure. The laboratory may do a screening test first, and then if that is positive do a quantitative measurement. Some laboratories will do the quantitative measurement directly. The quantitative measurement depends on the addition of a reagent which produces a purple color in the presence of 5-HIAA. The intensity of the color is then measured by a spectrophotometer.

Possible Interfering Materials and Conditions. There may be an elevated urinary excretion of 5-hydroxyindoleacetic acid in patients with non-tropical sprue, but this elevation is generally much less than that found in carcinoid.

The urine 5-HIAA levels may be increased if the patient has, in the preceding 3 days, eaten bananas, plantains, or certain other fruits not yet identified. The following drugs, listed by official (generic) name, may also produce increased levels if taken in the preceding 3 days:

Acetanilid	Methysergide maleate
Glyceryl guaiacolate	Phenothiazines
Mephenesin	Reserpine
Methocarbamol	

The urinary 5-HIAA levels may be artifically depressed

if the patient has received one of the phenothiazine-type drugs (see table 25).

Normal Range:

For screening test—negative.

For quantitative measurement—2 to 10 mg. in 24 hours.

17 Hydroxy Corticosteroids (Also Known as 17 Hydroxysteroids Abbreviated as 17-OHCS)

This is primarily a test of adrenal cortex function. The adrenal cortex produces corticosteroids which are altered and then excreted largely in the urine. The level of 17 hydroxy corticosteroids therefore may give an indication of the rate at which the adrenals are producing the corticosteroids. In cases of hyperadrenalism (Cushing's syndrome) the urinary levels are higher than normal. However, the reverse is not necessarily true. In cases of hypoadrenalism the urinary levels of 17 hydroxy corticosteroids may be within the normal range. If adrenal cortical underfunction is suspected, but the urinary levels of 17-OHCS are normal, the physician may administer ACTH and retest the urinary 17-OHCS excretion. If adrenal cortical function is normal, the urinary excretion of 17-OHCS will rise markedly after ACTH. However, if adrenal cortical function is poor, the urinary levels of 17-OHCS will not rise much.

Food and Drink Restrictions. None.

Procedure for Collecting Specimen. Place a large clean urine collection container in the refrigerator. Collect each urine sample from the patient during a 24-hour period in a regular clean urine bottle and pour it into the large refrigerated container. During the 24-hour collection period, the patient should drink 6 to 8 glasses of fluids.

Laboratory Procedure. The 17-OHCS are extracted from the urine with butanol, and a phenylhydrazine-sulfuric acid reagent is added. The resulting color change is measured by spectrophotometer.

Possible Interfering Materials and Conditions. Many drugs interfere with this test, and it is advisable to avoid administering any medications to the patient for at least 3 days before the test. It is of some interest that while cortisone and several of its derivatives tend to elevate the urinary levels of 17-OHCS, some of the high-potency derivatives, such as dexamethasone tend to decrease the urinary levels. Apparently, the reason for this effect of dexamethasone is that by inhibiting ACTH production, it causes a diminution of adrenal cortical secretion, while its own breakdown products are low in quantity because of low dosage. Some of the substances known to interfere with this measurement are the following, listed by official (generic) name:

Acetazolamide
Chloral hydrate
Chlordiazepoxide
Chlormerodrin
Chlorothiazide
Chlorpromazine
Colchicine
Corticosteroids
Cortisone
Dexamethasone
Dextroamphetamine
Digitoxin
Digoxin
Estrogens
Ethinamate
Glutethimide
Hydralazine
Hydroxyzine
Iodides
Meprobamate
Oleandomycin
Oral contraceptives
Paraldehyde
Penicillin
Perphenazine
Phenazopyridine
Phenothiazines
Piperidine
Prochlorperazine
Promazine
Quinidine
Quinine
Reserpine
Spironolactone
Testosterone
Triacetyloleandomycin

Normal Range. 4 to 14 mgm. in 24 hours. With other laboratory procedures, the normal range may differ.

Immunologic Test For Pregnancy

This test, developed rather recently, appears to be highly accurate. It has the advantages over the older pregnancy tests such as Aschheim-Zondek, Friedman, and Hogben in that it does not require the use of live animals and that a result is obtained in a shorter time. The immunologic test in sensitive enough to be positive in most cases of pregnancy by the 13th day after the first missed period (41 days after the onset of the last menstrual period). Since the test is based on the presence of chorionic gonadotropin in the urine, it will also be positive in cases of chorionepithelioma and hydatidiform mole.

Food and Drink Restrictions. None.

Procedure for Collecting Specimen. Any urine specimen may be used provided it is not grossly contaminated and does not contain blood. However, more concentrated specimens (specific gravity over 1.015) provide more accurate results.

Laboratory Procedure. A drop of urine is placed on a slide, a drop of antiserum to chorionic gonadotropin added, and mixed well for 30 seconds. Then, 2 drops of prepared antigen (latex particles coated with human chorionic gonadotropin) are added and mixed gently. If agglutination of the latex particles occurs within 2 minutes, the test is negative. If there is no agglutination within 2 minutes, the test is positive.

Possible Interfering Materials and Conditions. Chorionepithelioma and hydatidiform mole may produce positive test results.

Normal Range: In the absence of pregnancy, the test is negative.

17 K

See 17-Ketosteroid Excretion.

17 Ketosteroid Excretion

The 17-ketosteroids are male hormones with a ketone group on the 17th carbon atom of the phenanthrene ring. In men two-thirds of these hormones are produced by the adrenals and only one-third by the testes. In women virtually all of these materials are secreted by the adrenals. Accordingly, it should be clear that, although they are male hormones, the level of 17-ketosteroid excretion is usually more important in diagnosing disorders of the adrenals than disorders of the testes.

In children the level of 17-ketosteroids is normally very low. Low levels of these compounds are found in adrenal hypofunction from any cause, including Addison's disease, myxedema, pituitary hypofunction and many types of severe debilitating illness.

High levels of 17-ketosteroids are found in certain types of adrenal or testicular hyperfunction. In women with virilizing syndromes, the 17-ketosteroid excretion is usually moderately elevated.

Very marked elevations, over 100 mg. a day, suggest either carcinoma of the adrenal cortex or the extremely rare interstitial cell tumor of the testis.

Food and Drink Restrictions. None.

Procedure for Collecting Specimen. Into a large bottle, usually of gallon size, 3 cc. of acetic acid is placed as a preservative. The patient's urine for a 24-hour period is then collected in this bottle. If the patient has been receiving bicarbonate of soda, a greater amount of acetic acid might be required to maintain the acidity of the specimen. The specimen should be kept refrigerated.

Laboratory Procedure. One method in common use is the measurement, colorimetrically, of the intensity of a red color produced when M-dinitrobenzene is added.

Possible Interfering Materials and Conditions. The 17-ketosteroid level may be elevated if the patient has taken one of the following drugs, listed by official (generic) name:

Chlordiazepoxide	Penicillin
Cortisone	Phenothiazines (table 25)
Ethinamate	Spironolactone
Meprobamate (table 23)	Triacetyloleandomycin
Oleandomycin	

The 17-ketosteroid level may be decreased if the patient has received any of the following:

Chlorothiazide	Piperidine
Cortisone derivatives of high potency	Quinidine
	Quinine
Methyprylon	Secobarbital
Paraldehyde	Thiazides
Phenazopyridine	

The test procedure may be interfered with by many drugs, making an accurate reading impossible. Such drugs include those listed above plus the following:

Betamethasone	Oral contraceptives
Dexamethasone	Probenecid
Estrogens	Pyrazinamide

Normal Range:
Men, 8 to 20 mg. per day;
Women, 5 to 15 mg. per day.

Lead

In suspected lead poisoning the determination of lead concentration in the urine may aid in diagnosis.

Food and Drink Restrictions. The patient must be on a low calcium diet for at least 3 days before the test to mobilize the lead from the bones.

Procedure for Collecting Specimen. Collect a 24-hour specimen in a special large bottle.

Laboratory Procedure. Both chemical and spectrographic methods are available. The latter method is preferred and is based on the absorption of specific wavelengths of light by the lead.

Possible Interfering Materials and Conditions. None reported yet.

Normal Range. Under 100 micrograms per 24 hrs.

Melanin

This test is an aid in the diagnosis of melanoma. Melanin

or its precursor, melanogen, appears in the urine in this disease but is also found in several other conditions. Melanin colors the urine brown or black. Melanogen is colorless.

Food and Drink Restrictions. None.

Procedure for Collecting Specimen. A urine sample is placed in a bottle and sent to the laboratory.

Laboratory Procedure. To a sample of urine is added sodium nitroprusside and sodium hydroxide. If a deep red color appears, glacial acetic acid is added and the instant production of a blue color indicates melanogen.

Possible Interfering Materials and Conditions. None reported yet.

Normal Range. Normally there is no melanin or melanogen in the urine.

Melanogen

See Melanin.

Microscopic Tests

Microscopic examination of the urinary sediment may reveal important information about the condition of the urinary tract. Red blood cells in males, or in females who are not of menstrual age, suggest bleeding somewhere along the tract, from glomerulus to urethra. When red blood cells are found, further studies are usually performed to determine the exact source of the blood. White blood cells (pus cells) in males or in catheterized specimens from females suggest infection of the urinary tract. Casts in the urine suggest some disorder of the kidney tubules. Crystals of certain kinds (sulfonamide) may indicate a need for change in therapeutic regimen.

Food and Drink Restrictions. None

Procedure for Collecting Specimen. A urine specimen is placed in a bottle and sent to the laboratory.

Laboratory Procedure. A sample of the urine is centrifuged and the sediment examined microscopically.

Possible Interfering Materials and Conditions. None reported yet.

Normal Range. Normally there are not more than two or three red blood cells per high power field, and very few white blood cells in the urine of males. In urine of females of menstrual age, substantial quantities of both red and white blood cells may be found. A few casts may be present normally, but large numbers of casts suggest kidney disease.

Morphine

This test is performed to determine whether the patient has taken morphine or heroin during the preceding 24 hours. (Heroin is metabolized to morphine in the body.) Its usual use is in methadone maintenance programs for heroin addicts, to see if the patient is abstaining from heroin. The test for urine morphine is positive only if the patient has taken morphine or heroin within the previous 24 hours. Hard-core heroin addicts who are being treated by methadone maintenance are, for months or years, completely unreliable and untrustworthy, and therefore objective tests are needed to monitor their progress.

Food and Drink Restrictions. None.

Procedure for Collecting Specimen. The urine specimen must be collected under the direct observation of a member of the clinic or hospital staff who actually sees the patient urinate into the container, and who then takes the container from the patient. Under no circumstances can the patient be trusted when he states that a sample is his, or that it was passed at a particular time.

If a urine sample is collected daily (7 times a week), one can be sure of the validity of the results. However, if a urine sample is collected and analysed less frequently, there must be a completely randomized and unpredictable pattern of collection days, so that when the patient arrives at the clinic, he does not know if a urine sample will be required or not. If a clinic requires a urine test only 5 days a week, some patients may revert to heroin on Friday evening and Saturday, confident that their urine specimens from Monday through Friday will be negative. If a clinic has a randomized collection program, it should be arranged so that Saturdays and Sundays are included in the pattern.

No special preservatives are needed for the urine.

Laboratory Procedure. The morphine is identified by thin layer chromatography.

Possible Interfering Materials and Conditions. None reported yet.

Normal Range. Normally, there is no morphine in the urine.

Myoglobin

Myoglobin is a normal constituent of muscle, similar in some respects to hemoglobin. In some conditions in which severe muscle destruction occurs, the myoglobin leaks out of the muscle, into the blood and thence to the urine. It is quite soluble in an alkaline urine, but if the urine is acid, the myoglobin may precipitate in the kidney tubules, blocking them and causing kidney damage. In severe cases, the kidney damage can be fatal. The most striking example is the so-called "crush syndrome" in which large muscle masses (usually the thigh) are crushed in an accident, and myoglobin appears in the urine. Myoglobinuria in lesser degree also occurs in dermatomyositis, after eating fish which have been poisoned by factory wastes, and in other conditions of muscle destruction. Myoglobin colors the urine brown or red.

Food and Drink Restrictions. None.

Procedure for Collecting Specimen. A urine sample is placed in a bottle and sent to the laboratory.

Laboratory Procedure. There are several procedures available. A positive benzidine test (*see* P.145) of the urine indicates that either myoglobin or hemoglobin is present. To differentiate between these two, several methods may be used. A differential precipitation with ammonium sulfate can be done without special equipment. If a reversion spectroscope or spectrophotometer is available, they may be used.

Possible Interfering Materials and Conditions. None reported yet.

Normal Range. Normally, no myoglobin is found in the urine.

17-O.H.

See 17 Hydroxy Corticosteroids

17-O.H.C.S.

See 17 Hydroxy Corticosteroids

pH

This is a measure of the degree of acidity or alkalinity of the urine. The kidney maintains the blood at the correct pH by excreting into the urine any excess ions which might alter the pH of the blood. The urinary pH, therefore, varies widely and changes do not indicate abnormality. However, in certain situations it is advisable to have an acid or alkaline urine and the pH measurement is important. When sulfadiazine is administered or when there is marked hemolysis or destruction of muscle tissue (crush syndrome), an alkaline urine is needed to keep the excreted substances soluble. Sulfadiazine, and the products of hemolysis and muscle destruction, are quite soluble in an alkaline urine, but in acid urine they precipitate and may cause urinary blockage and death. In treatment with certain urinary tract antiseptics (methenamine) an acid urine is needed. In bladder infections the urine may be highly alkaline because bacteria transform urea into ammonia.

Food and Drink Restrictions. None.

Procedure for Collecting Specimen. A urine specimen is placed in a bottle and sent to the laboratory. In infants treated with sulfadiazine, the urinary pH is important, but collection of a urine sample may be difficult. A simple expedient is to place a strip of nitrazine paper inside the diaper at each change. The pH of the urine is then determined by the color of the nitrazine paper at the next diaper change.

Laboratory Procedure. A strip of nitrazine paper is dipped into the urine. The color change, compared to a standard chart, indicates the pH. A pH meter may be used.

Possible Interfering Materials and Conditions. None reported yet.

Normal Range. pH 4.8 to 8.0.

Phenolsulfonphthalein (P.S.P.) Test

This is a test of the ability of the kidney tubules to excrete a dye. The urinary excretion of injected phenolsulfonphthalein is decreased in chronic nephritis and urinary tract obstructions. It may be increased in certain liver diseases.

Food and Drink Restrictions. None.

Procedure for Collecting Specimen. It is not necessary for the patient to empty the bladder before beginning the test. The patient drinks two glasses of water. Thirty minutes later, the physician injects 1 cc. of phenolsulfonphthalein intravenously. Urine specimens are then collected in separate containers at intervals of 15, 30, 60 and 120 minutes after injection of the dye and sent to the laboratory.

Laboratory Procedure. The urine samples are alkalinized to bring out the maximum color and compared to standards in a colorimeter.

Possible Interfering Materials and Conditions. In liver disease, there may be a spurious increase in phenolsulfonphthalein excretion.

In multiple myeloma and hypoalbuminemia, there may be a spurious decrease in phenolsulfonphthalein excretion.

The P.S.P. levels may be elevated by several drugs. Those currently known, listed by official (generic) name, include:

Anthraquinone derivatives	Danthron
Cascara	Ethoxazene

Novobiocin

Phenazopyridine drugs
(see table 17)

Phenolphthalein

Probenecid

Pyridium

Radiographic contrast
media

Rhubarb extracts

The P.S.P. readings may be decreased by the following:

Diuretics

Penicillin

Salicylates (see table 27)

Sulfonamides

Normal Range. Elimination of 63 to 84 per cent of the injected dye in 2 hours. For greater sensitivity the percentage excreted in each fraction is calculated.

Phenylketonuria Test

This test is designed to uncover early cases of phenylketonuria (phenylpyruvic oligophrenia). In this condition the patient—an infant—is unable to metabolize phenylalanine, an essential amino acid, properly. As a result, pathologic metabolic end products are formed which lead to permanent mental deficiency. If the disorder is recognized early, a phenylalanine deficient diet can be given and the mental deficiency avoided. Accordingly, it is important to recognize the disorder as soon as possible. In some hospitals a routine diaper test is performed on all infants over 4 weeks of age, since infants with this disorder excrete phenylpyruvic acid in the urine after the age of 3 weeks.

In many states, the law requires that every infant be tested for phenylketonuria between the fourth and tenth weeks of life. At least two urine tests, a week apart, are required. Positive results must be reported to the Board of Health.

A blood test (see P. 75) is useful at ages as low as three days, so that it is being used instead of the urine test in many hospitals.

Food and Drink Restrictions. None.

Procedure for Collecting Specimen. Several pieces of absorbent or filter paper are placed in the baby's diaper by the mother or nurse. After they have been wet with urine, they are dried and sent to the laboratory.

Laboratory Procedure. A dried paper strip is tested with a drop of 10% ferric chloride solution. If phenylpyruvic acid is present the paper turns green, and the green color fades in 5 minutes. If the test is positive or doubtful, more precise chemical tests can be performed on the other papers for confirmation.

Possible Interfering Materials and Conditions. The phenylketonuria test may be interfered with if the patient has received chlorpromazine, aspirin or other salicylates (table 27) since ferric chloride produces a pink color with metabolites of these drugs.

Normal Range. Normally there is no phenylpyruvic acid in the urine, and the test is negative.

Porphyrins

Porphyrins are pigments, similar to bilirubin, and probably come from the hemoglobin of the blood. Normally there is an insignificant amount of porphyrin in the urine. In certain conditions, such as toxic liver damage, lead poisoning, some blood disorders, pellagra, and congenital porphyria the urinary excretion of porphyrins rises.

Food and Drink Restrictions. None.

Procedure for Collecting Specimen. The total urine excreted by the patient over a 24-hour period is collected in a large bottle. The sample should be kept refrigerated.

Laboratory Procedure. The urine is treated so as to precipitate and concentrate any porphyrins which may be present. The redissolved precipitate is examined spectroscopically for the absorption bands characteristic of porphyrins.

Possible Interfering Materials and Conditions. The urine porphyrin level may be increased if the patient has received one of a number of drugs. The list, by official (generic) name, includes:

Acriflavine	Penicillin
Alcohol	Phenazopyridine
Antipyretics	Phenothiazines (see
Barbiturates (see table 18)	table 25)
Chloroquine	Phenylhydrazine
Chlorpromazine	Procaine
Ethoxazene	Sedatives and hypnotics
Oxytetracycline	Sulfonamides

Normal Range. A minute quantity may normally be found in the urine.

P.S.P.

See Phenolsulfonphthalein Test

Slide Test For Pregnancy

See Immunologic Test for Pregnancy

Specific Gravity

This measurement indicates the degree of concentration of dissolved material in the urine. Ordinarily the specific gravity rises when the fluid intake is low and falls when fluid intake is high. In certain kidney disorders involving the tubules the urine is not concentrated or diluted beyond relatively narrow limits.

Food and Drink Restrictions. None.

Proceduce for Collecting Specimen. A urine sample is placed in a bottle and sent to the laboratory.

Laboratory Procedure. The extent to which a standard urinometer sinks in the urine determines the specific gravity.

Possible Interfering Materials and Conditions. The specific gravity may be increased if the patient has received dextran or radiographic contrast media.

Normal Range. 1.003 to 1.030.

Sugar

See Fermentation Test for Sugar

Sugar, Qualitative

In some disorders sugar is found in the urine. This occurs most often in diabetes mellitus, but may also occur in other metabolic disorders of varying importance. Because of its simplicity this test is usually employed as a screening procedure to discover diabetes. If sugar is found, other tests may then be ordered to determine the type of sugar (*see Fermentation Test for Sugar*).

Food and Drink Restrictions. None.

Procedure for Collecting Specimen. A urine sample is placed in a bottle and sent to the laboratory.

Laboratory Procedure. The more complex tests of a few years ago have now been replaced with simplified tablet tests. A specified amount of urine is added to a tablet and the color produced indicates the presence or absence of sugar.

Possible Interfering Materials and Conditions. A large number of drugs may produce false positive tests for sugar in the urine. Sometimes the type of test procedure used by the laboratory may make a difference. The drugs reported able to produce false positive, or spurious elevations in urine sugar levels, listed by official (generic) name, include:

Acetanilid	Corticosteroids
Aminosalicylic acid	Diatrizoate
Antipyrine	Edathamil
Ascorbic acid (large doses)	Ephedrine, large doses
Aspidium oleoresin	Ethacrynic acid
Bismuth salts	Gluconates
Carinamide	Indomethacin
Cephalothin	Isoniazid
Chloral hydrate	Metaxalone
Chloramphenicol	Nalidixic acid
Chlortetracycline	Nicotinic acid
Cinchophen	Nitrofurantoin

Nitrofurazone
Para-aminosalicylic acid
Penicillin
Phenacetin
Probenecid
Pyrazolone derivatives
Quinethazone

Salicylates (table 27)
Streptomycin
Sulfonamides
Tetracyclines
Thiazides
Trioxazine
Vaginal powders, some

Normal Range. Normally there is no sugar in the urine.

Sugar, Quantitative

This test is performed on some diabetics to determine the extent of sugar loss.

Food and Drink Restrictions. None.

Procedure for Collecting Specimen. A 24-hour urine specimen is collected in a clean bottle and sent to the laboratory. The specimen should be kept refrigerated, and preserved with some toluol.

Laboratory Procedure. A sample of the urine is titrated with Benedict's quantitative solution. The disappearance of color from the Benedict's solution marks the end point.

Possible Interfering Materials and Conditions. A large number of drugs may produce false positive tests for sugar in the urine. Sometimes the type of test procedure used by the laboratory may make a difference. The drugs reported able to produce false positive, or spurious elevations in urine sugar levels, listed by official (generic) name, include:

Acetanilid
Aminosalicylic acid
Antipyrine
Ascorbic acid (large doses)
Aspidium oleoresin
Bismuth salts
Carinamide
Cephalothin
Chloral hydrate

Chloramphenicol
Chlortetracycline
Cinchophen
Corticosteroids
Diatrizoate
Edathamil
Ephedrine, large doses
Ethacrynic acid
Gluconates

Indomethacin
Isoniazid
Metaxalone
Nalidixic acid
Nicotinic acid
Nitrofurantoin
Nitrofurazone
Para-aminosalicylic acid
Penicillin
Phenacetin

Probenecid
Pyrazolone derivatives
Quinethazone
Salicylates (table 27)
Streptomycin
Sulfonamides
Tetracyclines
Thiazides
Trioxazine
Vaginal powders, some

Normal Range. Normally there is no sugar in the urine.

Sulkowitch Test

See Calcium Test (Sulkowitch)

Thorn Test

See Chapter 7

Urea Clearance

This test is seldom performed these days because it has been replaced by less cumbersome, more useful tests of kidney function.

Urobilinogen

This is a test to aid in the differential diagnosis between complete and incomplete obstruction of the biliary tract. Increases in urinary urobilinogen (a breakdown product of hemoglobin) occur in many conditions, including hemolytic diseases, liver damage and severe infections. However, in complete obstructive jaundice without infection there is ordinarily no excess of urobilinogen in the urine.

When antibiotics are being administered, this test may not be accurate. Antibiotics inhibit growth of intestinal bacteria, and therefore interfere with the production of urobilinogen in the intestine.

Food and Drink Restrictions. None.

Procedure for Collecting Specimen. Place 5 gm. of sodium carbonate in a brown glass bottle and keep in refrigerator, avoiding unnecessary exposure to light. A urine sample is placed in the bottle, and sent to the laboratory. In some institutions, a random sample of urine may be used; in others a 2-hour morning specimen or a 24-hour urine may be tested.

Laboratory Procedure. To serial dilutions of the urine sample is added Ehrlich's reagent. The greatest dilution giving a pink color is determined. Labstix are also available for rapid diagnosis.

Possible Interfering Materials and Conditions. The urobilinogen level may be falsely elevated if the patient has received any of the following materials (asterisk indicates official or common name):

Amidopyrine	*Phenazopyridine
*Antipyrine	(see table 17)
*Bromsulphalein (B.S.P.)	Pyradone
*Chlorpromazine	Pyramidon
*Diatrizoate	Pyridium
Hypaque	Thoradex
*P-Aminosalicylic acid	Thorazine
Novocaine	

Urobilinogen levels may be reduced if the patient has received an antibiotic or chemotherapeutic agent which affects the microorganisms in the intestine.

Normal Range. A positive reaction at a urine dilution of not more than 1:20. This corresponds to a maximum excretion rate of 4 mgm. in 24 hours by an adult.

Vanilmandelic Acid (VMA)

This is a test for pheochromocytoma (see Catecholamines, P. 147) Pheochromocytoma is a rare tumor of the chromaffin cells of the adrenal medulla and other parts of the sympathetic nervous system. Such tumors secrete excessive amounts of catecholamines like epinephrine (Adrenalin) and arterenol. The metabolic breakdown of these catecholamines in the body results in several products, of which vanilmandelic acid (VMA) is the most prominent. Accordingly, the discovery of a high level of vanilmandelic acid in the urine may be an important aid to the diagnosis of pheochromocytoma.

Two related tumors, neuroblastoma and ganglioneuroblastoma, found mainly in infants and young children, also produce elevated urinary levels of vanilmandelic acid.

This is a rather non-specific test, and may give false positive results unless closely correlated with clinical observations of the patient's signs and symptoms.

Food and Drink Restrictions. Certain foods and beverages are believed capable of producing phenoxyacids in the urine, and these may give false results. Accordingly, such items must be omitted for at least 3 days before the test, and during the collection of the urine.

At our present level of knowledge, the foods and beverages to be omitted are chocolate, coffee, tea, vanillin, and all fruits. It is likely that other dietary items will also be found to interfere with this test.

Procedure for Collecting Specimen. The patient should take no drugs for 3 days before the beginning of the test. Notify the laboratory that the test has been ordered. Place 10 cc. of *concentrated* hydrochloric acid in a large bottle for a 24-hour urine specimen. Observe precautions to avoid spattering any of the acid on persons or materials. If possible, obtain a prepared bottle from the laboratory. Make sure there is no acid on the outside. Place all urine voided during 24 hours in the large bottle.

Laboratory Procedure. The vanilmandelic acid is extracted from the urine and oxidized to vanillin. The vanillin is extracted and measured spectrophotometrically.

Possible Interfering Materials and Conditions. Many foods and drugs are known to interfere with vanilmandelic acid measurements, and others will probably be added to the list in the future. For this reason, all drugs should, if possible, be discontinued at least 3 days before the test and during the collection of the urine sample.

Foods and beverages that may give spuriously elevated urine vanilmandelic acid levels include:

Bananas   Tea
Chocolate   Vanilla flavoring
Coffee

Drugs that may give spuriously elevated urinary vanil-mandelic acid levels include (asterisk indicates either the common or the generic name):

°Anileridine   °Methenamine
°Cough medicines (some)   °Methocarbamol
°Glyceryl guaiacolate   Robaxin
 Leritine   °Salicylates (see table 27)
 Mandelamine   Tolserol
°Mephenesin

In addition, reserpine derivatives (table 26) may interfere with the reading of vanilmandelic acid levels.

Normal Range. The normal amount of vanilmandelic acid in a 24 hour urine specimen is not more than 7 mg.

VMA

See Vanilmandelic Acid

d-Xylose Tolerance Test (Oral)

This is a test of the ability of the gastrointestinal tract to absorb nutrients. There are several disorders of absorption which, if accurately diagnosed, can be corrected by appropriate treatment.

The d-xylose is ordinarily absorbed by the gastrointestinal tract and then excreted by the kidney. If, after ingestion, the amount found in the urine is low (assuming kidney function is adequate), it is probable that a disorder of gastrointestinal absorption exists. The d-xylose is used instead of glucose because several conditions may produce misleading absorption figures with glucose.

Food and Drink Restrictions. The patient must fast overnight before the test. Water is permitted as desired.

Procedure for Collecting Specimen. Urine is voided and discarded. Then, 25 Gm. of d-xylose are mixed with 500 cc. of water and swallowed. After one hour an additional 250 cc. of plain water is taken, and another hour later, another 250 cc. All urine is collected for 5 hours from the ingestion of the d-xylose. At least 150 cc. of urine must be voided and collected.

Laboratory Procedure. A sample of urine is heated with a special reagent mixture which changes the xylose into a pink-colored material. The intensity of the color is compared to a standard in a colorimeter.

Possible Interfering Materials and Conditions. There may be a reduction in d-xylose excretion if the patient has taken isocarboxazid (Marplan) or phenelzine (Nardil).

Normal Range. 5 to 8 Gm. of d-xylose in the urine in 5 hours (20 to 32 per cent absorption).

6

Tests Performed on Feces

Although relatively few tests are done on feces, those which are performed are important to the patient whose health or life may depend on an accurate diagnosis based on such an examination. Careful collection and handling of the specimen and expert, conscientious performance of the examination are as essential as in any other test.

Blood

The discovery of blood in the feces may uncover a serious bleeding lesion of the gastrointestinal tract. Blood from a lesion in the lower colon is bright red and readily recognized. However, blood coming from the stomach or small intestine is so changed by the digestive process that it is not recognizable on inspection. Therefore, chemical tests are performed to see if there is occult blood in the feces.

Food and Drink Restrictions. Food restrictions vary. See next paragraph.

Procedure for Collecting Specimen. Sometimes, any random stool is used. At other times, since meat may also give a positive result, the physician may order the test after the patient has been on a meat-free diet for 3 days. On a meat-free diet, poultry and fish should also be omitted.

Laboratory Procedure. To the stool is added either benzidine or guaiac. A blue color represents a positive result.

Possible Interfering Materials and Conditions. There may be a false positive reaction for occult blood in the feces if the patient has taken any of the following:

> Bromides
> Iodides (see table 22)
> Iron-containing medications

Meat, poultry, fish

It should also be noted that pyrvinium pamoate (Povan) stains stools red, so that there may be the appearance of frank bleeding. However, the staining is harmless.

Even on a meat-free diet, some people will normally show a positive test if their gums bleed when the teeth are brushed.

Normal Range. On a regular diet, many persons normally have positive benzidine or guaiac tests.

Fat Determination

This test is used to confirm the diagnosis of steatorrhea (excess fat in the stools). The steatorrhea itself may be the result of pancreatic disease, obstruction of the biliary tract, interference with intestintal absorption, conditions which block the intestinal lymphatics, or sprue.

Food and Drink Restrictions. The patient should be on a normal diet for at least 3 days before the sample is collected.

Procedure for Collecting Specimen. A sample of feces at least 5 Gm. in weight is placed in a container and sent to the laboratory. In some institutions, a two or three day sample of feces is used.

Laboratory Procedure. The feces sample is dried and weighed. The fat is extracted with a solvent which is subsequently evaporated. The fat which remains is then weighed.

Possible Interfering Materials and Conditions. None reported yet.

Normal Range. Between 15 and 25 per cent of the weight of the fecal sample.

Parasites

Examinations of feces for parasites are performed in order to identify the parasites or their eggs. The therapy will usually depend on the type of parasite found, so that precise identification is important.

Food and Drink Restrictions. None.

Procedure for Collecting Specimen. The sample of feces is obtained and kept in various ways, depending on the type of parasite sought. Oily cathartics are never given. An ordinary "cold" stool is suitable for examination for ova and for amebic and similar cysts. A "warm" stool, which is kept at approximately body temperature until delivery at the laboratory, is suitable for all the previous examinations and also for trophozoites (mobile forms). A proctoscopic aspiration or scraping may be tested for trophozoites. A proctoscopic biopsy may be done for Schistosoma ova. Anal swabs are done for pinworm eggs. All samples are brought to the laboratory at once.

Laboratory Procedure. The stool samples are examined microscopically and parasites and ova identified.

Possible Interfering Materials and Conditions. None reported yet.

Normal Range. A large percentage of the population harbors harmless parasites like E. coli and certain flagellates.

Undigested Food

The finding of large amounts of undigested food may indicate some abnormality of digestion.

Food and Drink Restrictions. None.

Procedure for Collecting Specimen. A stool specimen is placed in a container which is covered tightly.

Laboratory Procedure. The specimen is examined macroscopically and, if requested, chemical tests for starch and fat may be performed.

Possible Interfering Materials and Conditions. None reported yet.

Normal Range. There is usually a small residue of undigested food in all feces.

Urobilin

Normally there are considerable amounts of urobilin

(also called stercobilin) in the feces. However, in complete obstruction of the bile passages, the feces contain no urobilin and are lighter than usual, often clay colored. This test may be useful in diagnosing complete biliary obstruction and in ascertaining when the obstruction becomes partially relieved.

Food and Drink Restrictions. None.

Procedure for Collecting Specimen. A stool specimen is placed in a container which is covered tightly.

Laboratory Procedure. A sample of the feces is mixed with a saturated solution of mercuric chloride. Urobilin will produce a deep red color after an interval of 6 to 24 hours.

Possible Interfering Materials and Conditions. None reported yet.

Normal Range. There is usually considerable urobilin in the feces.

7

Miscellaneous Tests

The following tests do not fall into any of the preceding categories. They measure important aspects of body function.

Basal Metabolic Rate (B.M.R.)

This test gives an indication of the rate at which metabolic processes take place under standard conditions. The basal metabolic rate may be elevated in such conditions as hyperthyroidism, anxiety and infection. It may be lowered in hypothyroidism and during sedation.

Although the B.M.R. is being replaced by other tests, it remains useful in many situations when properly performed.

Food and Drink Restrictions. The patient must fast for at least 10 hours before the test. Water may be taken ad lib.

Procedure for Performing Test. The patient, from the outset, must understand the test procedure thoroughly since any anxiety about it might change the basal metabolic rate. He should have a good night's sleep before the test. In the test the patient lies on a comfortable cot and breathes pure oxygen. The BMR machine records the amount of oxygen used per unit of time. From this the basal metabolic rate is calculated.

Possible Interfering Materials and Conditions. Almost any drug can affect the basal metabolic rate.

Normal Range. —20 to +20 per cent.

Biopsy

Biopsies are examinations of tissue specimen removed from the patient. They may be performed on many kinds of tissue from almost any area. Biopsies may be done to help diagnose various conditions, including malignancies.

182

Food and Drink Restrictions. None.

Procedure for Collecting Specimen. The doctor removes the specimen, using whatever technique is appropriate. A biopsy is a surgical procedure requiring strictest precautions.

Laboratory Procedure. The tissue specimen is fixed, sectioned, stained and examined microscopically by a pathologist. In some cases, in order to save time, examination of a frozen section may be performed.

Possible Interfering Materials and Conditions. None reported yet.

BMR

See Basic Metabolic Rate

Breath Alcohol

As a result of the highway accident toll, breath alcohol measurements are now being performed on automobile drivers who are suspected of being drunk, or who have been involved in a serious accident. Ordinarily, a member of a police unit performs the test, and is specially trained to do so.

No one can be forced to submit to a test of breath alcohol. However, if a driver refuses to take the test, he automatically loses his license in most states. If he wishes to do so, a driver may ask that a physician draw a sample of his blood for a test (see P. 34).

The breath alcohol test has proven to be a reliable measurement of blood alcohol concentration, and there is little chance of its being in serious error despite any maneuvers of the subject.

Blood levels of alcohol under 0.05% mean that the subject is not legally considered to be under the influence of alcohol. However, even such low levels reduce driving ability significantly. Levels between 0.05% and 0.15% may or may not be considered to mean that the subject is under the influence of alcohol, depending on other evidence. Levels of 0.15% and over are considered clear evidence of being under the influence of alcohol. At levels of 0.25% and over, there is marked intoxication and beginning stupor. At about 0.40%, coma occurs, and at slightly higher levels, death can result.

Food and Drink Restrictions. The subject must wait at least 15 minutes after his last drink of an alcoholic beverage before taking the test. This precaution is necessary to prevent a falsely high reading from traces of alcohol in the mouth. If he wishes, the subject may rinse his mouth with plain water (not mouthwash) before the test, but this is not necessary. If the subject has eaten, or drunk non-alcoholic beverages such as tea or coffee between the time of ingesting alcohol and the time of testing, the results will not be significantly affected.

Procedure for Collecting Specimen. All instruments now on the market have disposable mouthpieces for each subject, so there need be no fear of infection. The operator gets the machine ready, and when told to do so, the subject blows into the mouthpiece. The machine utilizes the latter part of the exhaled air, which is considered alveolar air.

In some cases, the police officer may not have a testing machine available, so the subject is asked to blow into a special balloon which is then sealed and sent to a laboratory for analysis.

Laboratory Procedure. Special machines are used for this particular procedure. There are several on the market. Standard solutions in ampuls are used, and the ability of alcohol in the breath to change the color is measured photoelectrically. The machines are calibrated in terms of blood alcohol percentage.

Possible Interfering Materials and Conditions. Methyl alcohol (wood alcohol) and isopropyl alcohol can produce measurable levels, but they are more toxic than ethyl alcohol.

Normal Range. Normally there is no alcohol in the blood or breath.

Capillary Fragility

See Tourniquet Test for Capillary Fragility

Chloride in Sweat

This is a test for cystic fibrosis of the pancreas. It has been found that children with cystic fibrosis excrete much greater amounts of chloride in their perspiration than do normal children. Therefore, if an excessively high concentration of chloride is found in the sweat, the presumptive diagnosis becomes cystic fibrosis, and the child is treated accordingly.

Some institutions use this test in a simplified form as a routine screening test in all children. It is hoped that the test will uncover early cases which can then be treated more effectively.

Food and Drink Restrictions. None.

Procedure for Performing Test. The child's hands are washed and dried. They are then kept from contact with other parts of the body for 15 minutes. After that interval a test paper, impregnated with silver chromate, is moistened with distilled or tap water (*not* saline), and the patient's hand is pressed down on the paper for 4 seconds. The print is then compared to that of a normal child. Whenever chloride is present, the red silver chromate changes to white silver chloride. The imprint of the normal child's hand is indistinct, while the imprint of the hand of the child with cystic fibrosis is heavy and distinct.

Possible Interfering Materials and Conditions. None reported yet.

Normal Range. Hand print is light and indistinct.

Diatrizoate Absorption Test

This test is used for early diagnosis of a perforation of the gastrointestinal tract. Its principal use is in accident cases, in which the doctor needs to know whether there has been a traumatic rupture. Diatrizoate is a substance which is not significantly absorbed by the normal gastrointestinal tract. However, it is rapidly absorbed from the peritoneal cavity and then excreted in the urine. If diatrizoate is administered to a patient without any gastrointestinal perforation, it will pass through the gut and be excreted in the feces; no significant amount will be excreted in the urine. On the other hand, if there is a gastrointestinal perforation, the diatrizoate will leak out into the peritoneal cavity, be absorbed, and be excreted in the urine.

The specific gravity of the material is high. Therefore, it tends to move down the gastrointestinal tract rapidly even if peristalsis is absent provided the patient's position is suitable. Furthermore, since it is a radiopaque contrast medium, its location in the GI tract can readily be determined by x-ray or fluoroscopy.

Although this is a relatively new test, it appears to have considerable promise in the early diagnosis of gastrointestinal perforation, before the classical signs of peritonitis are seen. It is reported to be more accurate than the radiologic technique of searching for air under the diaphragm.

Diatrizoate is available under several brandnames, including Hypaque, Gastrografin, Cardiografin, and Renografin.

Food and Drink Restrictions. When perforation is suspected, the patient should receive neither food nor water by mouth.

Procedure for Performing the Test. A urine sample is obtained from the patient, by voiding or catheterization.° The specific gravity is measured, and three drops of concentrated hydrochloric acid added slowly. No precipitate should be seen. If a precipitate is seen, the patient has probably been receiving large doses of penicillin.

The patient is then given 30 to 50 cc. of diatrizoate by

°Since the risk of gastrointestinal perforation is far greater than the risk of a urinary tract infection, there need be no hesitation about catheterizing these patients.

mouth. Movement of these patients may be dangerous, since there could be other injuries. Accordingly, the nurse should not attempt to change the patient's position. This should be done by the physician or under his direct observation.

Urine samples are taken every 15 minutes for several hours. For each specimen, the specific gravity is first measured, and then three drops of concentrated hydrochloric acid are added.

If no precipitate forms, the chances of there being a gastrointestinal perforation are reduced.

If a thick, chalky white precipitate forms, and was not produced in the control urine, the presumptive diagnosis is gastrointestinal perforation.

If a precipitate is noted in both control and later urines, the specific gravities are compared. If the specific gravity of the urine after administration of diatrizoate exceeds 1.040, the presumptive diagnosis is gastrointestinal perforation, since diatrizoate produces such elevations in specific gravity, while other chemicals, such as penicillin which can also cause precipitation do not.

This test is always an emergency test, and the urine examinations should be done and reported immediately.

Possible Interfering Materials and Conditions. Large doses of penicillin may result in a urinary precipitate after acidification, but the comparison of urine specific gravities should provide the correct diagnosis.

Normal Range. Normally, no precipitate of diatrizoate will occur in the urine.

Electrocardiogram (E.C.G.)

The electrocardiogram records the electrical potentials produced by the heart. All cells possess bioelectricity. Very sensitive instruments can pick up a difference of potential between the inside and outside of any living cell. With muscle and nerve cells, following stimulation, the cell membrane becomes permeable to certain ions, and a current flows between the inside and outside of the cell. The difference in potential travels as a wave down the cell. Our knowledge of the exact mechanisms involved is still incomplete, although most scientists believe they consist of depolarization and repolarization of the cell membrane. The electrocardiograph is a sensitive instrument, recording the changes in electrical potential of the heart which are transmitted through the limbs and chest wall. The record itself is called the *electrocardiogram*. It should be noted that only electrical potentials are measured. These electrical potentials are not directly related to force of contraction. Therefore, the electrocardiogram gives no indication as to the strength of the heart. In fact, it is possible, experimentally, to record a normal-looking electrocardiogram from a heart so weakened that no contraction whatever can be observed or recorded. The electrocardiogram is useful in diagnosing cardiac arrhythmias and in diagnosing and following the course of myocardial infarctions. Electrocardiograms are interpreted by cardiologists.

Food and Drink Restrictions. None.

Procedure for Performing Test. Appropriate electrodes are strapped to the patient's limbs and chest and connected to the machine which records the tracing. There are many varieties of electrocardiographs and each is operated somewhat differently from the others.

Possible Interfering Materials and Conditions. A number of drugs, including the cardiac glycosides affect the electrocardiogram. The significance of such effects is determined by the cardiologist.

Normal Range. The cardiologist decides whether the tracing is normal.

Electroencephalogram (E.E.G.)

This is a record of the electrical potentials produced by the brain cells. It may be used in the diagnosis of epilepsy and similar disorders. It is far more complex than the electrocardiogram. The electrical potentials which are recorded from the brain may be 100 times weaker than those recorded by the electrocardiogram, so that a much more sensitive instrument (electroencephalograph) is required to record them. Special precautions must be taken against electrical interference.

Food and Drink Restrictions. None.

Procedure for Performing Test. Electrodes are fastened to the patient's scalp and connected to the machine which records the tracing.

Possible Interfering Materials and Conditions. A number of drugs, including sedatives, may affect the EEG. The neurologist determines the significance of such effects.

Normal Range. The neurologist decides whether the tracing is normal.

G.A.

See Gastric Analysis

Gastric Analysis (Tube)

This test is performed to determine the degree of acidity of stomach contents. It is an uncomfortable procedure for most patients, so that newer tests of gastric acidity, using various resins, have been devised.

The stomach ordinarily secretes hydrochloric acid to aid in digestion. In certain conditions, such as duodenal or gastric ulcer, the quantity of acid may be greater than normal. In other conditions, such as pernicious anemia, gastric carcinoma and simple achlorhydria, there may be none of the acid. Occasionally, the gastric contents may be examined for enzymes, tissue fragments and tubercle bacilli.

Food and Drink Restrictions. The patient receives nothing by mouth after supper on the night before the test, unless ordered by the doctor.

Procedure for Collecting Specimen. The physician coats a cold Levin tube with mineral oil, inserts it into the patient's mouth or nose, and passes it down the esophagus into the stomach. An emesis basin is always kept at hand since some patients become nauseated. After insertion of the Levin tube the physician sucks out the stomach contents with a large syringe, and subsequently stimulates gastric secretion. This may be done by feeding the patient a test meal or by injecting histamine or betazole hydrochloride (Histalog). Some patients develop severe reactions to these injected materials, and may lose consciousness. Therefore, any patient receiving an injection to augment gastric secretion should be observed *continuously* until the test is completed. In addition, epinephrine, aqueous solution, 1:1,000, and a syringe and needle should be ready on a tray, and 0.3 to 0.5 cc. injected intramuscularly if necessary.

Laboratory Procedure. The samples of gastric juice are first tested for free hydrochloric acid and then for total hydrochloric acid content, including that bound to other substances. In each case the gastric juice sample is titrated with sodium hydroxide in the presence of reagents which change color at specific pHs.

Possible Interfering Materials and Conditions. None reported yet.

Normal Range. With histamine, usually 100 to 160 degrees of acidity, but 8 per cent of healthy persons have no acid. The normal range depends on the type of stimulus used to induce gastric secretion. The total acidity is usually up to 20 degrees greater than the free acidity. A degree of acidity represents the number of cc. of 1/10 normal sodium hydroxide needed to neutralize 100 cc. of gastric juice. It is also equivalent to 3.65 mg. of hydrochloric acid.

Gastric Analysis (Tubeless)

This method of determining the presence of stomach acid does not require the passing of a tube into the esophagus and is more comfortable for the patient. It is based on the fact that free hydrochloric acid will displace certain materials from combination with other subtances. The earlier tubeless analyses were performed with quininium resin indicator. More recently, an azure indicator dye has been used.

In general this method is not suitable for exact quantitative analysis but gives the essential information needed in many cases, i.e., whether free acid is present in the stomach. Since false negative reactions sometimes occur, a negative report is not diagnostic of achlorhydria unless confirmed by standard gastric analysis. The tubeless method can save most patients from the discomfort of intubation.

Food and Drink Restrictions. No food is taken after midnight, but water is permitted as desired.

Procedure for Collecting Specimen. In the morning, the first urine specimen is discarded. The patient is then given a glass of water with 500 mg. of caffeine sodium benzoate. After one hour he urinates, and the urine specimen is saved as a control. He then swallows the blue granules of the dye in one-half glass of water. After an additional 2 hours he urinates, and the urine is sent to the laboratory. The urine may be blue or green for several days after. This has no significance.

Laboratory Procedure. Both urine specimens are diluted to 300 cc., and 10 cc. aliquots are compared to standards.

Possible Interfering Materials and Conditions. In patients who have had such operations as subtotal gastrectomy, gastroenterostomy, or pyloroplasty, both false negative and false positive results may occur. In patients with malabsorption syndrome, severe diarrhea, pyloric obstruction, severe liver disease, severe kidney disease, severe dehydration, or urinary retention, the results of this test may be misleading.

The diagnex blue level may be falsely elevated if the patient has taken the following within the preceding 2 days (asterisk indicates either the official or the common name):

*Aluminum
*Antacid medications
Atabrine
*Barium
*Calcium
Cremomycin
Donnagel

*Iron
*Kaolin
Kaopectate
*Magnesium
*Methylene blue
*Nicotinic acid
Pomalin

°Potassium, large amounts   °Riboflavin
°Quinacrine   °Sodium, large amounts
°Quinidine   °Vitamin B capsules
°Quinine

In addition, phenazopyridine (table 17) which colors the urine orange may make it impossible to obtain any reading.

Normal Range. A blue color equal to or more than 0.6 mg. standard indicates the presence of free hydrochloric acid in the stomach.

Gastrointestinal Perforation

See Diatrizoate Absorption

Microscopic Tests for Malignant Cells (Papanicolaou Smear)

In many areas of the body malignant (cancer) cells separate from tumors and may be identified microscopically. This may make possible the diagnosis of malignancy early enough for satisfactory treatment or even complete cure. Such tests are most commonly performed on the female genital tract but are also of value in other areas. Other specimens include bronchial, esophageal, rectal, and colonic washings, duodenal drainage, gastric and nipple secretions, pleural, peritoneal and pericardial exudates, prostate smears, sputum and urine.

Food and Drink Restrictions. None.

Procedure for Collecting Specimen. The physician collects the specimen. If it consists of a washing, drainage, exudate, aspiration fluid or urine, it is mixed with equal parts of 95% alcohol and sent to the laboratory. If it consists of a smear or a secretion, it is smeared on a glass slide which is then immersed in a solution containing equal parts of 95% alcohol and ether *before the smear can dry.* Sputum is collected in 70% alcohol. Other types of fixing solutions are also available, and may be used for some specimens.

Laboratory Procedure. The fluid specimens are concentrated by centrifugation and smeared. All smears are stained and examined microscopically.

Normal Range. No malignant cells are found normally.

Papanicolaou Smear

See above

Pregnancy Tests

See Chapter 5

Radioiodine Uptake

This test has become a major tool in diagnosis of thyroid conditions. It is based on the fact that the radioactive isotope of iodine, I^{131}, is taken up by the thyroid in the same manner as ordinary iodine. The breakdown of I^{131} to more stable elements results in the release of gamma rays which can be detected and counted by a scintillation counter held near the patient's neck. The degree of radioactivity is a measure of the degree of iodine uptake. Uptake below normal ranges suggests hypothyroidism; above normal ranges suggests hyperthyroidism. It has been estimated that this test is performed on 1,000 patients per day. The amount of radioactivity involved is too small to harm the patient, and much too small to be a hazard to anyone else. This test should be distinguished from the use of radioiodine *in therapy,* where much larger amounts are used.

Food and Drink Restrictions. None.

Procedure for Performing Test. No special preparation is necessary. The patient's past history must be checked for any excess iodine consumption which would give misleading test results. If the patient has taken any of the drugs listed in table 22, within a 30-day period, that information should be given to the radiology laboratory at once. If the patient has had x-ray studies of the gallbladder, uretes, bronchi, fallopian tubes, heart or other organs in which iodinated contrast media were used, that information should be noted, even if many years have elapsed. If the patient has eaten large amounts of sea food in the previous 2 weeks, that fact too should be noted. Where necessary, the patient may be reassured that the amount of radioactivity involved is too small to do any real harm. Furthermore, it can be pointed out that I^{131} has a short half-life (8 days) so that it will disappear, rapidly. The patient can continue normal food and water intake. A capsule containing the radioactive iodine is swallowed by the patient. After exactly 24 hours, the amount of radioactivity coming from the thyroid gland is measured in the radiology laboratory, using a scintillation counter. Sometimes, 24-hour urines are also collected and measured for radioactivity. After the test is completed, the patient may be given some Lugol's solution, or other medication containing regular iodine. This will displace most of the remaining radioactive iodine from the body.

Possible Interfering Materials and Conditions. If the patient has received during the preceding 30 days any of the iodine-containing drugs listed in table 22 there may be a misleading depression of radioiodine uptake. Some breads in which iodides are used as dough conditioners may also cause lower readings. In addition, other drugs that can depress the radioiodine uptake, listed by official (generic) name, include:

ACTH
Antihistamines
Butazolidin
Chlordiazepoxide
Chlortetracycline
Cortisone (see table 20)
Diazepam
Methimazole
Methylthiouracil
Nitrates
Para-aminosalicylic acid
Penicillin
Phenothiazines (see table 25)
Phenylbutazone
Sulfonamides
Testosterone
Thiopental
Thiouracil
Thyroglobulin
Thyroid, dessicated
Thyronine
Thyroxine

A misleading elevation of the radioiodine uptake may be produced by estrogens (see table 21).

Normal Range. Radioactive iodine uptake of 20 to 40 per cent.

Rumpel-Leede Test

See Tourniquet Test for Capillary Fragility

Schilling Test

This is a test for pernicious anemia and related conditions. Patients with pernicious anemia and certain other disorders cannot absorb cyanocobalamin (Vitamin B_{12}) properly. Therefore, when radioactive cyanocobalamin is given orally, and followed by intramuscular non-radioactive cyanocobalamin, the excretion of radioactive cyanocobalamin in the urine is less than normal. The test is usually given in stages. If the first stage shows a normal urinary excretion of cyanocobalamin, pernicious anemia is probably not present, and the test is terminated. But if the first stage shows a lower than normal urinary excretion of radioactive cyanocobalamin, a second, and possibly a third stage of testing may be needed to rule out conditions other than pernicious anemia that can cause decreased gastrointestinal absorption of cyanocobalamin.

Stage 1

Food and Drink Restrictions. The patient must fast for at least 12 hours before the test and during the test until he receives the injection of non-radioactive cyanocobalamin. Water is permitted.

Procedure for Collecting Specimen. The patient voids and the urine is discarded. Then 0.5 microcuries of radioactive cyanocobalamin are swallowed. From this point on, all urine is collected for 24 hours and stored. No special preservatives or refrigeration are needed for the urine, but complete collection is vital.

Two hours after taking the radioactive cyanocobalamin orally, the patient receives 1 mg. of non-radioactive cyanocobalamin by intramuscular or intravenous injection. (Some authorities recommend that this be given 30 minutes rather than 2 hours after the oral administration. Check with the laboratory as to the method preferred.)

The patient may eat after the injection of non-radioactive cyanocobalamin.

If stage 1, of this test shows a lower than normal excretion of radioactive cyanocobalamin in the urine (under 7%), stage 2 is performed.

Stage 2

It is advisable to wait 5 days after stage 1 before performing stage 2, although in some institutions the wait may be shorter.

Food and Drink Restrictions. The patient must fast for at least 12 hours before the test and during the test until he receives the injection of non-radioactive cyanocobalamin. Water is permitted.

Procedure for Collecting Specimen. The patient voids and the urine is discarded. Then, 0.5 microcuries of radioactive cyanocobalamin are swallowed, plus 60 milligrams of intrinsic factor from pigs. From this point on, all urine is collected for 24 hours and stored. No special preservatives or refrigeration are needed for the urine, but complete collection is vital.

Two hours after taking the radioactive cyanocobalamin orally, the patient receives 1 mg. of non-radioactive cyanocobalamin by intramuscular or intravenous injection. (Some authorities recommend that this be given 30 minutes rather than 2 hours after the oral administration. Check with the laboratory as to the method preferred.)

The patient may eat after the injection of non-radioactive cyanocobalamin.

If stage 2 of this test shows an excretion of over 7% of the radioactivity in 24 hours, and if stage 1 showed less than 7%, the probable diagnosis is pernicious anemia. If, however, both stages 1 and 2 show a 24 hour excretion of radioactivity under 7%, stage 3 is performed.

Stage 3

Stage 3 is carried out to discover whether an alteration in the bacteria of the intestine is interfering with absorption of cyanocobalamin and producing signs and symptoms similar to pernicious anemia. Stage 3 requires 11 days for completion.

Food and Drink Restrictions. For the first 9½ days of this stage of the test, there are no restrictions. But the patient must fast for at least 12 hours before the administration of the cyanocobalamin and continue to fast during the test until he receives the injection of non-radioactive cyanocobalamin. Water is permitted.

Procedure for Collecting Specimen. For 10 days, the patient receives tetracycline, 250 mg. four times daily by mouth (to reduce the bacteria in the gastrointestinal tract.) At the end of this period, the procedure described for stage 1 is repeated.

If the excretion of radioactivity after stages 1 and 2 had been less than 7%, and if after stage 3 it is more than 7%, the probable diagnosis is bacterial interference with cyanocobalamin absorption.

Laboratory Procedure. The radioactivity of an aliquot of the urine is measured in a scintillation counter.

Possible Interfering Materials and Conditions. Therapeutic doses of cyanocobalamin given in the 3 days preceding the test may interfere with interpretation of the results.

Kidney disease may cause a deceptively low excretion of the radioactivity during the test period. In such cases, a prolonged testing period may be required.

Normal Range. Normally, the 24-hour excretion of radioactive cyanocobalamin in stage 1 is greater than 7% of the amount ingested.

Sputum Smears for Eosinophiles and Elastic Fibers

The sputum contains eosinophiles in cases of allergic

asthma, but not in "cardiac" asthma. Finding eosinophiles may, therefore, aid in the differential diagnosis between these two conditions. If elastic fibers are found in the smear, there is probably a destructive lesion of the walls of the alveoli or bronchioles, such as tuberculosis with cavitation, malignancy, or lung abscess.

Food and Drink Restrictions. None.

Procedure for Collecting Specimen. Sputum is collected in a container which is then covered. In some institutions the sputum is smeared on 2 slides in the patient's room. Elsewhere, the smearing is done in the laboratory.

Laboratory Procedure. The slides are stained and examined microscopically for eosinophiles and elastic fibers.

Possible Interfering Materials and Conditions. None reported yet.

Normal Range. Normally there are very few, if any, eosinophiles or elastic fibers in the sputum.

Thorn Test

This test, named after its originator, is a test of adrenal function. There are two parts. At times, both parts taken together are called *the* Thorn test. Some doctors, on the other hand, refer to 2 separate Thorn tests—the Thorn Eosinophile test, and the Thorn Uric Acid Excretion test. Therefore, if a Thorn test is ordered, it is advisable to determine exactly which one is meant.

When the adrenals are unable to perform their function, as in Addison's disease, they do not respond to injections of ACTH (adrenocorticotrophic hormone from the pituitary). Persons with normal adrenal function respond to injections of ACTH by a decrease in the circulating eosinophiles and by a marked rise in the excretion of uric acid as compared to creatinine. Patients with Addison's disease do not show such changes.

Food and Drink Restrictions. The patient must fast for 12 hours before the test. Water may be taken as desired.

Procedure for Collecting Specimen. There are marked

variations between hospitals in the procedures used, so that the following is a general guide only. A urine sample is collected over a measured time interval and sent to the laboratory. A technician also performs eosinophile counts on the peripheral blood. Then the physician injects ACTH, either in a single injection or as an infusion over a period of hours. Urine samples are collected, marked with time of voiding, and sent to the laboratory. In addition, a technician performs one or more eosinophile counts on the peripheral blood.

Possible Interfering Materials and Conditions. None reported yet.

Normal Range:

Eosinophile level—in normal adrenal function, the eosinophile level drops by at least 50 per cent.

Uric acid excretion—in normal adrenal function, there is approximately a 100 per cent rise in uric acid excretion. In Addison's disease, the increase is usually below 20 per cent.

Thyrotropin Test (TSH)

This test is used in several situations in which the diagnosis of thyroid deficiency is difficult or complicated. Thyrotropin is the thyroid stimulating substance secreted by the pituitary gland. Under the influence of large doses of thyrotropin, the thyroid will secrete as much thyroid hormone as it can. The thyrotropin test is used mainly to distinguish primary hypothyroidism from hypothyroidism secondary to pituitary dysfunction. In primary hypothyroidism, the injection of thyrotropin will produce only a minimal increase in thyroid function, while in secondary hypothyroidism, the injection of thyrotropin will produce a major increase in thyroid function. If the patient has primary hypothyroidism, the protein-bound iodine level and the radioiodine uptake will be about the same after thyrotropin as before. If he has secondary hypothyroidism, the protein-bound iodine and radioiodine uptake will be significantly higher after thyrotropin than before. Also, in patients who have been taking thyroid medication without a definite diagnosis of hypothyroidism, the medication can obscure the findings of most of the relevant tests, but the thyrotropin test can sometimes help clarify the situation. Finally, in borderline cases of hypothyroidism, in which other tests of thyroid fuction give suggestive but not clear-cut results, the thyrotropin test results can sometimes help the physician make a definitive diagnosis.

Food and Drink Restrictions. None.

Procedure for Collecting Specimen. First, a regular radioiodine uptake and a protein-bound iodine test are performed (P.193 and P.105). Then, thyrotropin is injected. A single injection of 5 units 1.M. or S.C. is recommended by some authorities, while others suggest 3 injections of 5 units at 24-hour intervals. Twenty-four hours (other intervals used in some institutions) later, the radioiodine uptake and protein-bound iodine tests are repeated.

Laboratory Procedure. See Protein-Bound Iodine and Radioiodine Uptake

Possible Interfering Materials and Conditions. See Protein-Bound Iodine Radioiodine Uptake

Normal Range. The concept of a normal range is not relevant here.

Tourniquet Test for Capillary Fragility

This test measures the ability of the capillaries to remain intact under stress. Increased capillary fragility may be found in many types of systemic vascular abnormalities, including scurvy, thrombocytopenic purpura, and purpura accompanying severe infections.

Procedure for Performing Test: The physician inflates a blood pressure cuff on the patient's arm to a point midway between diastolic and systolic pressures. The pressure is maintained for 10 minutes. Any petechiae (small hemorrhages under the skin) render the test positive. Sometimes counts of petechiae per unit of area may also be reported.

Possible Interfering Materials and Conditions. None reported yet.

Normal Range. Some people will normally have a positive test, particularly those with red hair.

Xylose

See Chapter 5

8

Normal Values in Infants and Children

In infants and children the normal values for many laboratory tests differ considerably from those of adults. In the body of this book the values given are for adults. In this section, however, the important differences in the values for infants and children will be considered.

Blood

At birth, the infant usually has a higher hemoglobin content than the adult. The average is about 17 Gm. per 100 cc., but higher concentrations are normal. This high level falls rapidly. At the age of 2 months it is about 14 Gm. per 100 cc., and at about 3 months it reaches a low point of about 11 Gm. per 100 cc. Thereafter, the hemoglobin content tends to rise very slowly, reaching about 13 Gm. per 100 cc. at the age of 2 years.

The red blood cells follow a similar pattern.

The white blood cells (leucocytes) are very numerous at birth. They average 20,000 per cubic mm. of blood, but counts as high as 35,000 per cubic mm. are normal. This is about 4 times the adult level. The leucocyte count falls gradually but remains higher than the adult level for at least the first 2 years of life. Accordingly, an elevated leucocyte count in a young infant has little or no diagnostic significance.

The infant normally has some degree of icterus with an elevated serum bilirubin from the second day to the seventh. This results from two factors—a considerable degree of destruction of the red blood cells and immaturity of the liver.

On the other hand, an excessive degree of icterus or visible icterus within 24 hours of birth may denote a serious condition, such as erythroblastosis fetalis (*Chapter* 3: *Blood Types/Rh factor*) which requires prompt, efficient therapy.

In newborn infants a low fasting blood glucose, about 50 mg. per 100 cc., or sometimes even lower, is common. This rises gradually, reaching 75 mg. per 100 cc. in the small child.

The total cholesterol in newborn infants is quite low, ranging from 80 to 165 mg. per 100 cc. of blood. However, this level rises until, in most children, it reaches 200 to 300 mg. per 100 cc. This is higher than usual adult levels. It may not be a strictly physiologic change. There is a strong likelihood that the high serum cholesterol levels in American children result from their high intake of dairy products after the age of weaning.

The alkaline phosphatase levels are high, up to 20 Bodansky units because of the formation of new bone cells.

During the first few days of life the level of blood urea nitrogen may be as high as 40 mg. per 100 cc., of blood. However, it rapidly falls to the adult level.

In the newborn the blood potassium level may be as high as 7 milliequivalents per liter. It, too, soon drops to adult levels.

Urine

Albuminuria is a common, almost universal, finding in infants during the first week or two of life. In older children it may or may not indicate the presence of disease.

Infants and children under 8 years of age normally excrete practically no 17-ketosteroids. At the age of 8, excretion increases gradually, reaching adult levels at about age 18. Increased levels in infants and young children may result from adrenal hyperplasia.

Cerebrospinal Fluid

In the newborn the glucose levels in the cerebrospinal fluid may normally be as low as 35 mg. per 100 cc. This, of course, is correlated with the low blood glucose levels. As the blood glucose levels rise, so do the CSF levels.

9

Units of Measurement Used in Clinical Laboratory Procedures

A *gram* (Gm.) is a standard unit of weight or mass. It is equivalent to 1/28 ounce.

A *milligram* (mg., mgm.) 1/1000 of a gram.

A *microgram* (microgm., mcgm., gamma) is 1/1,000,000 of a gram.

A *milligram per cent* is a milligram per 100 cubic centimeters or per 100 grams.

A *cubic centimeter* (cc.) is a unit of volume equal to a cube 1 centimeter in each dimension. It is equivalent to a milliliter (1/1000 of a liter) for practical purposes.

A *cubic millimeter* (cubic mm.) is a unit of volume equal to a cube 1 millimeter in each dimension. It is equivalent to 1/1000 of a cubic centimeter for practical purposes.

A *liter* (1.) is a unit of liquid measurement. It is equivalent to 1000 cubic centimeters, or about 1 quart.

A *volume per cent* is a measurement of the amount of gas dissolved in a liquid. For example, when 10 cc. of gas is dissolved in 100 cc. of fluid, the concentration can be expressed as 10 volumes per cent.

A *mol is* the number of grams equal to the number expressing the molecular weight of the substance. Since sodium, for example, has a weight of 23, a mol of sodium is 23 grams.

A *molar* solution is a mol of a substance dissolved in enough fluid to make 1 liter of solution. Thus a molar solution of sodium has 23 grams of sodium per liter.
23 milligrams.

A *millimol* is 1/1000 of a mol. A millimol of sodium is

A *millimolar* solution is a millimol of a substance dissolved in enough fluid to make 1 liter of solution. A millimolar solution of sodium contains 23 milligrams of sodium per liter.

An *equivalent* is a mol divided by a valence. An equivalent of sodium is 23/1 or 23 grams. An equivalent of calcium (weight 40, valence 2) is 40/2 or 20 grams.

A *milliequivalent* (mEq.) is 1/1000 of an equivalent. A milliequivalent of sodium is 23 milligrams and a milliequivalent of calcium is 20 milligrams.

A *degree of acidity* is the amount of acid contained in 100 cc. of gastric juice which will just neutralize 1 cc. of 1/10 normal sodium hydroxide solution. A degree of acidity is equivalent to 3.65 mg. of hydrochloric acid. This unit of measurement is used in describing the acidity of gastric juice.

A *unit* is an arbitrary measurement used when no other means of measurement is satisfactory. Units are usually based on a particular bio-assay technique. The unit in one kind of test bears no relationship to the unit in another kind of test.

10

Technique of
Venipuncture, etc.

Technique of Venipuncture

In some institutions nurses may perform venipuncture, although it is usually done by the physician or laboratory technician. Usually the veins of the ventral aspect of the elbow are used. The operator should make sure that the light is suitable and that he or she will be working in a comfortable position. A tourniquet is placed around the arm above the elbow and tightened so as to produce a pressure higher than that in the vein but lower than the diastolic pressure. The radial pulse should be checked after the tourniquet has been applied. If the pulse cannot be felt, the tourniquet should be loosened. In selecting a vein, the deeper ones which can be palpated but not seen are usually more satisfactory than the more superficial ones. The latter tend to have thick coats and to roll away from the needle. After deciding on the site of venipuncture the skin is cleansed with 70% alcohol which is allowed to dry thoroughly to prevent the painful results of introducing alcohol into the tissues with the needle. That area, thereafter, is not touched with anything but the needle. The needle is pushed through the skin and the point advanced until it penetrates the vein. Most beginners make the mistake of pushing the needle too far, so that it goes entirely through the vein. When blood appears in the syringe tip, the angle of insertion is changed by depressing the syringe, and the needle is advanced a few millimeters into the lumen of the vein. The tourniquet is then released, and after some 10 seconds the blood is drawn into the syringe. After sufficient blood has been withdrawn, the needle is quickly taken out, and a sterile gauze sponge is placed over the venipuncture site. The patient immediately flexes his arm so that the gauze sponge exerts pressure on the vein, preventing the blood from oozing out of the opening. The patient is instructed to maintain this position for several minutes.

A 20-gauge needle is used for most venipunctures, unless the patient is a child. Smaller needles are less painful but the blood does not flow through them rapidly enough for most purposes. Venipuncture with needles larger than 20-gauge may be uncomfortable for many patients.

The sterilization of blood lancets is also important. Although these lancets merely pierce the skin to draw a drop of blood, they can transmit infection, including hepatitis. Re-usable lancets should be autoclaved between each usage. The older method of "sterilization" in alcohol is unreliable. A leading authority* states:

"The use of blood lancets or knife blade for obtaining small amounts of blood must be recognized, likewise, as a procedure not without risk. Dipping a blood lancet into alcohol and allowing it to dry, or wiping a knife blade with a pad moistened with alcohol should not be considered as a safe procedure until there is published information on the effect of alcohol on these viruses. At present, there is circumstantial evidence of epidemiological nature that such procedures may be unsafe."

Disposable Equipment

There are now available several types of disposable sterile equipment for drawing blood and other specimens. In general, the cost of these sterile, single-use materials is quite low compared to the *total* cost of employing reusable items which includes initial purchase, breakage and the labor needed to clean, package and sterilize for the next patient. Usually, the disposable items are as economical as the re-

---

*Reddish, G. F. *Antiseptics, disinfectants, fungicides, and chemical and physical sterilization.* Lea and Febiger, Philadelphia, 2nd Ed., 1957, p. 387.

usable ones, and in areas in which it is difficult to get hospital personnel, they are more economical. For this reason, many hospitals are shifting to disposable items.

The simplest type of disposable item consists of a single blade for finger-tip puncture.

There are two main types of disposable items for drawing venous blood. One consists of a disposable needle and disposable syringe. These are available as a single unit, or as two separate units.

Another device consists of a glass tube, with a rubber diaphragm stopper and a vacuum. It is used with a special double-ended needle. After one end of the needle is inserted into the lumen of the vein, the other end is pushed through the rubber stopper. The vacuum within the tube then draws in the correct amount of blood, and the test tube itself becomes the container for transporting the specimen to the laboratory. These tubes come in various sizes up to 30 ml., and with a variety of anticoagulants or none. The most commonly used brand is the Vacutainer. Tubes may be sterile or non-sterile depending on the test being performed. Apparently, it is believed that there is no risk from using a non-sterile tube in this situation, since the vacuum prevents any reflux of material back into the vein. If the Vacutainer tubes are used, one must be certain that the correct model tube is used for each specimen collected. At this time, there are scores of different combinations of tube sizes and anticoagulant types, identified by code numbers and stopper colors. Of course, many are interchangeable, and some are only used for relatively uncommon tests. The stopper colors cannot be used alone to identify the type of anticoagulant, since the same color may be used for more than one.

Selected References

Periodicals

Allen, R. J. and Wilson, J. L. Urinary phenylpyruvic acid in phenylketonuria. *J.A.M.A.*, *188*:720, 1964.

Alvarez, W. C. A great need for evaluating laboratory tests. *Modern Medicine*, April 1, 1958, p. 10.

Aring, C. D. An occupation for adults. *Arch. Int. Med.*, *116*:164, 1965.

Astin, T. W. Systemic reaction to bromsulphthalein. *Brit. Med. J.*, *2*:408, 1965.

Baer, D.M., and Krause, R. B. Spurious laboratory values resulting from simulated mailing conditions. *Am. J. Clin Path.*, *50*:111-119, 1968.

Barnett, R. N., Civin, W. H. and Schoen, I. Multiphasic screening by laboratory tests — an overview of the problem. *Am. J. Clin. Path.*, *54*:483-492, 1970.

Beeson, P. B. The case against the catheter. *Am. J. Med.*, *24*:1, 1958.

Behringer, B. R., and Stephenson, H. E., Jr. The diatrizoate precipitation test for intestinal perforation. *Surg., Gynec. & Obstet.*, *129*:475-482, 1969.

Berry, H. K., Sutherland, B., Guest, G. R. and Warkany, J. Simple method for detection of phenylketonuria. *J.A.M.A.*, *167*:2189, 1958.

Betson, C. Blood gases. *Amer. J. Nursing*, *68*:1010-1012, 1968.

Blum, N. I., Mayoral, L. G. and Kalser, M. H. Augmented gastric analysis — a word of caution. *J.A.M.A.*, *191*:339, 1965.

Borushek, S. and Gold, J. J. Commonly used medications that interfere

Briller, A. Important uses of electrocardiography. *Amer. J. Nursing*, *55*:1378, 1955 (Nov.).

Bronson, W. R., DeVita, V. T., Carbone, P. P. and Cotlove, E. Pseudohyperkalemia due to release of potassium from white blood cells during clotting. *New Eng. J. Med.*, *274*:369, 1966.

Caraway, W. T. Chemical and diagnostic specificity of laboratory tests. *Am. J. Clin. Path.*, *37*:445, 1962.

Castleman, B. Normal laboratory values. *New Eng. J. Med.*, *262*:84, 1960.

Charles, D., VanLeeuwen, L. and Turner, J. H. Significance of cornified cells in the vaginal smear of postmenopausal women. *Am. J. Obstet. Gynec.*, *94*:527, 1966.

Clark, M. B. Studies based on errors observed in the use of anticoagulants in blood chemistry determinations. *Am. J. Med. Technol.*, *17*:190, 1951.

Clarke, T. H. and Laipply, T. C. The use and abuse of laboratory tests in surgery. *Surg. Clin. N. America*, *44*:3, 1964.

Clayton, E. M., Altshuler, J. and Bove, J. R. Penicillin antibody as a use of positive direct antiglobulin tests. *Amer. J. Clin. Path.*, *44*:648, 1965.

Cohen, L. Serum enzyme determinations: Their reliability and value. *Med. Clin. N. America*, *53*:115-135, 1969.

Cranswick, E. H., Cooper, T. B. and Simpson, G. M. Two-year follow-up study of protein-bound iodine elevation in patients receiving perphenazine. *Am. J. Psychiat.*, *122*:300, 1965.

Croft, J. D., Jr., et al. Coombs'-test positivity induced by drugs. *Ann. Int. Med.*, *68*:176-186, 1968.

David, R. R., Alexander, D. S., and Wilkins, L. Placental transfer of an organic radiopaque medium resulting in a prolonged elevation of the protein-bound iodine. *J. Pediat.*, *59*:223-226, 1961.

Dawborn, J. K. and Plunkett, P. J. The collection and assessment of mid-stream urine samples in the diagnosis of urinary tract infection in women. *Med. J. Australia*, April 13, 1963, p. 540.

Didisheim, P. Tests of blood coagulation and hemostasis. *J.A.M.A.*, *196*:33, 1966.

Dlouhy, A., Erickson, Sr. M. B., Nedlicka, B., Imburgia, F., Ipavec, J. and Kiewlich, S. What patients want to know about their diagnostic tests. *Nursing Outlook*, *11*:265, 1963.

Editorial: Sterilization of syringes. *Canad. Med. Assn. J.*, *87*:138, 1962.

Editorial: The shrinking specificity of the transaminase determination. *J.A.M.A.*, *191*:101, 1965.

Editorial: Urinary phenylpyruvic acid in phenylketonuria. *J.A.M.A.*, *188*:748, 1964.

Elvebach, L. R., Guillier, C. L., and Keating, F. R., Jr. Health, normality, and the ghost of Gauss. *J.A.M.A.*, *211*:69-75, 1970.

Finlay, J. M., Hogarth, J. and Wightman, K. J. R. A clinical evaluation of the D-xylose tolerance test. *Ann. Int. Med.*, *61*:411, 1964.

Fisher, A. B., Levy, R. P. and Price, W. Gold — an occult cause of low serum protein-bound iodine. *New Eng. J. Med.*, *273*:812, 1965.

Fogel, B. J., Sanders, R. W., Fife, E. H. and Anderson, R. I. The serodiagnosis of early syphilis. How to utilize the newer laboratory tests. *Clin. Ped.*, *4*:447, 1965.

Foster, M. A. Teaching blood groups and reactions. *Nursing Outlook*, Feb. 1966, p. 49.

Foulk, W. T. and Fleisher, G. A. The effects of opiates on the activity of serum transaminase. *Proc. Staff Meet. Mayo Clin.*, 32:405, 1957.

Gault, M. H., and Dossetor, J. B. Editorial: The place of phenolsulfonphthalein (PSP) in the measurement of renal function. *American Heart J.*, 75:723-727, 1968.

Goldstein, A., and Brown, B. W., Jr. Urine testing schedules in methadone maintenance treatment of heroin addiction. *J.A.M.A. 311*-315, 1970.

Goldthwait, J. C., Butler, C. F. and Stillman, J. S. The diagnosis of gout. *New Eng. J. Med.*, 259:1095, 1958.

Grant, S. D., Foshman, P. H. and DiRaimondo, V. C. Suppression of 17-hydroxycorticosteroids in plasma and urine by single and divided doses of triamcinolone. *New Eng. J. Med.*, 273:1115, 1965.
with routine endocrine laboratory procedures. *Clin. Chem.*, 10:41, 1964.

Guze, L. B. and Beeson, P. B. Observations on the reliability and safety of bladder catheterization for bacteriologic study of the urine. *New Eng. J. Med.*, 255:474, 1956.

Hartney, J. B. The role of the clinical laboratory in the community hospital. *Med. Clin. N. America*, 53:11-23, 1969.

Haunz, E. A . The role of urine testing in diabetes detection. *Amer. J. Nursing*, 64:102, 1964 (Nov.).

Hayner, N. S., et al. Carbohydrate tolerance and diabetes in a total community, Tecumseh, Mich. *Diabetes*, 14:413, 1965.

Islam, M. A. and Sreedharan, T. Convulsions, hyperglycemia, and glycosuria from overdose of naldixic acid. *J.A.M.A.*, 192:1100, 1965.

Jackson, G. G. and Greeble, H. G. Pathogenesis of urine infection. *Arch. Int. Med.*, 100:692, 1957.

Kraus, S. J., Haserick, J. R., and lantz, M. A. Atypical FTA-ABS test flourescence in lupus erythematous patients. *J.A.M.A.*, 211:2140. 2141, 1970.

Kushner, D. S. Phenolsulfonphthalein excretion test. *J.A.M.A.*, 195: 1078, 1966.

Linton, K. B., and Gillespic, W. A. Collection of urine from women for bacteriological examination. *J. Clin. Path.* 22:376-380, 1969.

London, W. T., Vought, R. L. and Brown, F. A. Bread — a dietary source of large quantities of iodine. *New Eng. J. Med.*, 273: 381, 1965.

Luddecke, H. F. Basal metabolic rate, protein-bound iodine and radioactive iodine uptake: a comparative study. *Ann. Int. Med.*, 49: 305, 1958.

Mainwaring, C. Clean voided specimens for mass screening. *Amer. J. Nursing*, 63:96, 1963 (Oct.).

Mallin, S. R. and Gambescia, J. M. A fatal reaction to sulfobromophthalein. *J.A.M.A.*, 174:1858, 1960.

Marks, V. and Shackcloth, P. Diagnostic pregnancy tests in patients treated with tranquilizers. *Brit. Med. J.*, *1*:517, 1966.

Martin, M. M. New trends in diabetes detection. *Amer. J. Nursing*, *63*:101, 1963 (Aug.).

McBay, A. J. Carbon monoxide poisoning. *New Eng. J. Med.*, *272*:252, 1965.

McCraw, J. B., Mcleod, R. A. and Stephenson, H. E., Jr. A urine precipitation test for intestinal perforation. *Arch. Surg.*, *91*:248, 1965.

Merrett, D. A. and Sanford, J. P. Sterile voided urine culture. *J. Lab. Clin. Med.*, *52*:463, 1958.

Meyer, R. R. Effect of iopanoic acid on the sulfobromophthalein test. *J.A.M.A.* *194*:343, 1965.

Moertel, C. G., Beahrs, O. H., Woolner, L. B. and Tyce, G. M. Malignant carcinoid syndrome associated with noncarcinoid tumors. *New Eng. J. Med.*, *273*:244, 1965.

O'Leary, L. Electro-encephalography. *Amer. J. Nursing*, *55*:1238, 1955 (Oct.).

Oltman, J. E. and Friedman, S. Further report on protein-bound iodine in patients receiving perphenazine. *Amer. J. Psychiat.*, *121*:176, 1964.

Peters, T., Jr., and Davis, J. S. Serum heat-stable lactate dehydrogenase in the diagnosis of myocardial infarction. *J.A.M.A.*, *209*-1186-1190, 1969.

Pfeffer, R. B., Stephenson, H. E., Jr. and Hinton, J. W. The effect of morphine, demerol and codeine on serum amylase values in man. *Gastroenterology*, *23*:482, 1953.

Pierce, J. M., Jr., Ruzumna, R. and Segar, R. Standardization of the phenolsulfonphthalein excretion test in clinical practice. *J.A.M.A.*, *175*:711, 1961.

Questions and answers: Radioactive iodine test. *J.A.M.A.*, *168*:1731,
Questions and answers: Radioactive iodine test and steroids. *J.A.M.A.*, *168*:1734, 1958.

Reagan, J. W. Cytological studies. *Amer. J. Nursing*, *58*:1693, 1958.

Reznikoff, P. and Engle, R. L. The physician, the laboratory and the patient. GP, *26*:82, 1962.

Rivin, A. U. False endocrine test results due to drugs. *Calif. Med.*, *101*:283, 1964.

Russe, H. P. The use and abuse of laboratory tests. *Med. Clin. N. America*, *53*:223-231, 1969.

Sapira, J. D., Klaniecki, T., and Ratkin, G. Non-pheochromocytoma. *J.A.M.A.*, *212*:2243-2245, 1970.

Scardino, J. Lithium in affective disorders. *N.Y. State J. Med.*, *70*:638-642, 1970.

Schneider, E. M. Venous abnormalities following intravenous sodium sulfobromophthalein administration. *J.A.M.A.*, *194*:339, 1965.

Shapiro, R. and Man, E. B. Iophenoxic acid and serum-bound iodine values. *J.A.M.A.* *173*:1352, 1960.

Silberstein, E. B. The Schilling test. *J.A.M.A.*, *208*:2325, 2326, 1969.

Smith, F. E., Reinstein, H. and Braverman, L. E. Cork stoppers and hypercalcemia. *New Eng. J. Med.*, *272*:787, 1965.

Spangler, A. S., Jackson, J. H., Fiurmara, N. J. and Warthin, T. A. Syphilis with a negative blood test reaction. *J.A.M.A.*, *189*:87, 1964.

Stephenson, H. E., Jr., McCraw, J. and McLeod, R. Early diagnosis of abdominal trauma. *Missouri Med.*, *63*:267, 1966.

Stewart, M. J. Testing home tests for cervical cancer. *Amer. J. Nursing*, *65*:75, 1965 (Dec.).

Switzer, S. The clean voided urine culture in surveying populations for urinary tract infection. *J. Lab. Clin. Med.*, *55*:557, 1960.

Thompson, R. B., Mayo, R. W. and Bell, W. N. Critical evaluation of pregnancy tests. *Am. J. Clin. Path.*, *44*:585, 1965.

Watson, E. M. Clinical laboratory procedures. *Canadian Nurse*, *56*:881, 1960.

West, K. M. Laboratory diagnosis of diabetes — a reappraisal. *Arch. Int. Med.*, *177*:187, 1966.

Wilkinson, J. H. Clinical significance of enzyme activity measurements. *Clin. Chem.*, *16*:882-890, 1970.

Wirth, W. A. and Thompson, R. L. The effect of various conditions and substances on the results of laboratory procedures. *Am. J. Clin. Path.*, *43*:579, 1965.

York, P. S., Landes, R. R., and Seay, L. S. Coombs' positive reactions associated with cephaloridine therapy. *J.A.M.A.*, *206*:1086, 1968.

Books

Air Force Manual. *Laboratory Procedures in Blood Banking and Immunohematology.* A.F.M. 160-50, Dept. of Air Force, 1962.

Annino, J. S. *Clinical Chemistry Principles and Procedures,* 3rd edition. Boston: Little, Brown & Co., 1964.

Bauer, J. D., Ackermann, P. G., and Toro, G. *Bray's Clinical Laboratory Methods,* 7th edition. St. Louis: C. V. Mosby Co., 1968.

Behrendt, H. *Diagnostic Tests in Infants and Children,* 2nd edition. Philadelphia: Lea and Febiger, 1962.

Bennington, J. L., Fouty, R. A., and Hougie, C. *Laboratory Diagnosis.* London: Macmillan, 1970.

Davidsohn, I., and Henry, J. B. *Clinical Diagnosis by Laboratory Methods,*

14th edition. Philadelphia: W. B. Saunders Co., 1969.

Frankel, S., Reitman, S. and Sonnenwirth, A. C. *Gradwohl's Clinical Laboratory Methods and Diagnosis*, 6th edition. St. Louis: C. V. Mosby Co., 1963.

Lynch, M. L., Raphael, S. S., Mellor, L. D., Spare, P. D., and Inwood, M. J. H. *Medical Laboratory Technology and Clinical Pathology*, 2nd edition. Philadelphia: W. B. Saunders Co., 1969.

MacFate, R. P. *Introduction to the Clinical Laboratory*, 2nd edition. Chicago: Year Book Medical Publishers, 1966.

PART TWO

Tables

1 Tests of Blood Function and Blood Disorders

Test	Performed on
A/G ratio	Blood serum
Albumin	Blood serum
Bilirubin, partition	Blood serum
Bilirubin, total	Blood serum
Bleeding time	Capillaries of skin
Blood counts	Whole blood
Blood culture	Whole blood
Blood types	Whole blood
Calcium	Blood serum
Clotting time	Whole blood
CO_2 combining power	Blood serum
Coombs, Direct	Whole blood
Coombs, Indirect	Whole blood
Fibrinogen	Blood plasma
Globulin	Blood serum
Glucose-6-phosphate dehydrogenase	Red blood cells
Hematocrit	Whole blood
Hemoglobin	Whole blood
Hemoglobin electrophoresis	Red blood cells
Icterus index	Blood serum
Iron	Blood serum
Iron binding capacity	Blood serum
Magnesium	Blood serum
Malaria film	Whole blood
Methemoglobin	Whole blood
Partial thromboplastin time	Blood plasma
PCO_2	Whole blood
pH	Blood serum
Plasma electrophoresis for gammopathies	Blood serum
Platelet count	Whole blood
PO_2 (arterial)	Whole blood
Porphyrins	Urine

(Continued)

1   Tests of Blood Function and Blood Disorders

Test	Performed on
Potassium	Blood serum
Protein	Blood serum
Prothrombin time	Blood serum
Red cell fragility	Whole blood
Reticulocyte count	Whole blood
Schilling	Urine
Sedimentation rate	Whole blood
Sickle cell test	Whole blood
Sodium	Blood serum
Sulfhemoglobin	Whole blood
Tourniquet test for capillary fragility	Capillaries of skin of arm
Urinary blood	Urine

2   Tests of Liver Function and Liver Disorders

Test	Performed on
A/G ratio	Blood serum
Ammonia	Whole blood
Bilirubin, partition	Blood serum
Bilirubin, total	Blood serum
Bromsulphalein retention (B.S.P.)	Blood serum
Cephalin flocculation	Blood serum
Cholesterol	Blood serum
Cholesterol esters	Blood serum
Fecal urobilin	Feces
Glucose	Blood serum
Glucose tolerance	Blood serum and urine
Icterus index	Blood serum
Phosphatase, alkaline	Blood serum
Prothrombin time	Blood serum
Serum transaminase	Blood serum
Thymol turbidity	Blood serum
Urinary bile and bilirubin	Urine
Urobilinogen	Urine
Zinc sulfate turbidity	Blood serum

Test	*Performed on*
Addis	Urine
Albumin, globulin, A/G ratio and protein	Blood serum
Albumin (qualitative and quantitative) in urine	Urine
Calcium	Blood serum
Chlorides	Blood serum
CO_2 combining power	Blood serum
Concentration and dilution	Urine
Creatinine	Blood serum
Creatinine clearance	Urine and blood
Microscopic tests of urinary sediment	Urine
Non-protein nitrogen (N.P.N.)	Blood serum
Phenolsufonphthalein (P.S.P.)	Urine
Phosphorus	Blood serum
Potassium	Blood serum
Sodium	Blood serum
Specific gravity	Urine
Urea clearance	Blood serum and urine
Urea nitrogen	Blood serum

Test	Performed on
Acetone	Urine
Amino acids	Urine
Ammonia	Whole blood
Ascorbic acid	Blood plasma
Ascorbic acid tolerance	Blood
Ascorbic acid tolerance	Urine
Basal metabolic rate (B.M.R.)	Patient
Calcium	Blood serum
Carbon dioxide	Blood Plasma
Diacetic (aceto-acetic) acid	Urine
Fermentation test for sugar	Urine
Glucose	Blood serum
Glucose tolerance	Blood serum and urine
Guthrie	Whole blood
Homogentisic acid	Urine
Lipid fractions	Blood serum
Lipoprotein analysis	Blood serum
pH	Blood serum
Phenylketonuria	Urine
Radioiodine uptake	Patient
Sugar, qualitative and quantitative	Urine
Thyroxine iodine	Blood serum
Uric acid	Blood serum

5 Tests for infections, Microorganisms, and Resistance to Microorganisms

Test	Performed on
Agglutination	Blood serum
Anti-streptolysin O titer	Blood serum
Bacterial count, urine	Urine
Blood culture	Whole blood
C-reactive protein	Blood serum
Colloidal gold	Spinal fluid
Fluorescent antibody	Many substances
Fluorescent treponemal antibody absorption	Blood serum
Hepatitis test (blood)	Blood serum
Heterophile antibody	Blood serum
Latex slide agglutination	Blood serum
Malaria film	Whole blood
Miscellaneous fluid cultures	Body fluids
Nose and throat culture	Nose and throat secretions
Parasites	Stool
Sedimentation rate	Whole blood
Serological tests	Blood serum and spinal fluid
Special tests	Spinal fluid
Spinal fluid chlorides	Spinal fluid
Spinal fluid culture	Spinal fluid
Spinal fluid protein	Spinal fluid
Spinal fluid sugar	Spinal fluid
Sputum culture and smear	Sputum
Stool culture	Stool
Urine culture	Urine
White cell differential count	Whole blood
Wound culture	Wound exudates

6 Tests for Malignancy

Test	Type of Malignancy	Performed on
Aschheim-Zondek, quantitative	Teratoma	Urine
Bence Jones protein	Bone tumors	Urine
Catecholamines	Pheochromocytoma	Urine
5-Hydroxyindoleacetic acid	Carcinoid	Urine
Leucine aminopeptidase	Carcinoma of the pancreas	Blood serum
Melanin	Melanomas	Urine
Microscopic tests	All	Various fluids
Papanicolaou	All	Various fluids
Phosphatase, acid	Prostate carcinoma	Blood serum
Phosphatase, alkaline	Bone tumors	Blood serum
Vanilmandelic acid	Pheochromocytoma	Urine

7 Tests of Endocrine Glands and Their Function

Test	Gland	Performed on
Amylase	Pancreas	Blood serum
Amylase, urine	Pancreas	Urine
Calcium	Parathyroid	Blood serum
Calcium (Sulkowitch)	Parathyroid	Urine
Cholesterol, total	Thyroid	Blood serum
Glucose (sugar)	Pancreas	Blood serum and urine
Glucose tolerance	Pancreas	Blood serum and urine
17-Hydroxycortico-steroids	Adrenal cortex	Urine
Insulin tolerance	Pituitary and thyroid	Blood serum
17-ketosteroid excretion	Adrenal cortex	Urine
Lipase	Pancreas	Blood serum
Phosphorus	Parathyroid	Blood serum
Potassium	Adrenal cortex	Blood serum
Protein-bound iodine (P.B.I.)	Thyroid	Blood serum
Radioiodine uptake	Thyroid	Patient
Sodium	Adrenal cortex	Blood serum
Thorn	Adrenal cortex	Blood and urine
Thyrotropin	Thyroid	Blood serum

10   Tests Performed on Venous Blood

Test	cc. of blood	Acceptable Anticoagulants	Normal Range (Adults)
Heterophile antibody	5	None	Concentrations up to 1/28
Icterus index	5	None	4 to 6 units
Insulin tolerance	3 per Sample	Fluoride	Return to pre-injection level within 2 hrs.
Iron (serum)	20	None	90 to 150 microgm./100 cc. of serum in males. 70 to 130 microgm./100 cc. of serum in females
Iron-binding capacity	10	None	250 to 410 microgm./100 cc. of serum or plasma
Lactic dehydrogenase	4	None	150 to 500 B & B units (other units sometimes used, with different ranges)
Latex slide agglutination	5	None	Up to 1 to 40
Lead	10	Heparin, oxalate	0 to 50 microgm./100 cc. of blood
Leucine aminopeptidase	4	None	75 to 230 units/100 cc. of male serum 80 to 210 units/100 cc. of female serum
Lipase	6	None	1.5 units or less
Lipid fractions	20	None	See test
Lipoprotein analysis	4	None	Similar to standards
Lithium	6	None	None (See test for therapeutic range)
Lupus erythematosus cell (L.E.) test	5	Oxalate	None
Magnesium	5	None	1.7 to 2.8 mgm./100 cc. serum or 1.5 to 2.3 milliequivalents/liter
...hemoglobin	5	Oxalate, sodium citrate	None
...-protein nitrogen (N.P.N.)	5	Oxalate	15 to 35 mg./100 cc. of s...
...al thromboplastin	4.5	Special oxalate solution	Varies with laboratories
...ne (arterial)	Filled tube	Heparin	31 to 45 mm. mercury

(Co...

8   Tests for Poisoning

Test	Performed on
Carbon monoxide	Whole blood
Alcohol	Blood serum and breath
Barbiturates	Blood serum
Lead	Whole blood and urine
Methemoglobin	Whole blood
Porphyrins	Urine
Salicylates	Blood serum
Sulfhemoglobin	Whole blood

9   Miscellaneous Tests

Test	Performed on
Aschheim-Zondek	Urine
Chloride in sweat	Sweat
Congo red retention	Blood serum
Creatine phosphokinase	Blood serum
Diatrizoate absorption	Urine
Electrocardiogram (E.C.G.)	Patient
Electroencephalogram (E.E.G.)	Patient
Fecal blood	Feces
Fecal fat	Feces
Friedman (pregnancy)	Urine
Frog (pregnancy)	Urine
Gastric analysis	Gastric juice
Heat stable lactic dehydrogenase	Blood serum
Heroin (see morphine)	Urine
Hogben (pregnancy)	Urine
Immunologic test for pregnancy	Urine
Lactic dehydrogenase	Blood serum
Lithium	Blood serum
Lupus erythematosus cell test (L.E.)	Whole blood
Morphine	Urine
Myoglobin	Urine
Sulfonamide level	Blood serum
Transaminase (G.P.)	Blood serum
Urinary chlorides	Urine
d-Xylose tolerance (oral)	Urine

221

Test	cc. of blood	Acceptable Anticoagulants	Normal Range (Adults)
A/G ratio (see Albumin)			
Agglutination	5	None	See test
Albumin, globulin, protein, A/G ratio	6 (total)	None	3.2 to 5.6 Gm./100 cc. 1.3 to 3.2 Gm./100 cc. 6.0 to 8.0 Gm./100 cc. 1.5:1 to 2.5:1
Alcohol	10	None	None
Ammonia	5	Oxalate, E.D.T.A., heparin	Less than 75 microgm./100 cc. of blood
Amylase	6	None	80 to 150 units (Somogyi)
Anti-streptolysin O titer	5	None	Up to 166 Todd units./cc. of serum
Ascorbic acid	6	Oxalate, heparin	0.6 to 1.6 mg./100 cc. of plasma
Barbiturate	5	None	None
Bilirubin	5	None	0.1 to 1.0 mg./100 cc. of serum
Blood types	5	None	
Blood urea nitrogen (B.U.N.) (See Urea nitrogen)			
Bromsulphalein (B.S.P.)	5	None	Less than 0.4 mg./100 cc. of serum
Calcium	6	None	9.0 to 11.5 mg./100 cc. of serum
Carbon dioxide	to fill tube	Heparin	22 to 34 mEq./L. or 50 to 60 Vol. %
Carbon monoxide	5	Oxalate	Less than 0.8 vol. %
Cephalin flocculation	5	None	0 to 1+
Chlorides	5	None	100 to 106 mEq./L. of serum, or 355 to 376 mg. chloride/ 100 cc. of serum
Cholesterol	5	None	120 to 260 mg./100 cc. of serum
Cholesterol esters	7	None	60% to 80% of total cholesterol

(Continued)

Test	cc. of blood	Acceptable Anticoagulants	Normal Range (Adults)
Clotting time	4	None	According to method
CO_2 combining power	7	Heparin—or test tube with oil	53 to 78 volumes/100 cc. of serum or 24 to 35 millimoles/ liter of serum
Congo red retention	6	None	Less than 40% disappears from blood in 1 hr.
Coombs' Direct			Negative
Coombs' Indirect	2		
Creatine phosphokinase	5		Several minor blood groups
C-reactive protein	4	None	According to method
Creatinine	5	None	None
Fibrinogen	6	None	0.6 to 1.3 mg./100 cc. 200 to 600 mg./100 cc. pl
Fluorescent treponemal antibody absorption	5	Oxalate, heparin, E.D.T.A. None	Negative
Globulin (see Albumin)			
Glucose	3-5	Oxalate, heparin, so- dium fluoride, E.D.T.A.	80 to 120 mgm./100 serum or 70 to 105 cc. of whole blood
Glucose-6-phosphate dehydrogenase	4	Heparin	Substantial amounts
Glucose tolerance (oral)	3 per sample	Oxalate, heparin, so- dium fluoride, E.D.T.A.	Peak under 150 m serum. (May be a mgm. % for elder
Glucose tolerance (intravenous)	3 per sample	Oxalate, heparin, so- dium fluoride, E.D.T.A.	Return to fastin 1 hr.
Heat stable lactic dehydrogenase	6	None	Under 115 u
Hematocrit	4	Oxalate, heparin, E.D.T.A.	Men, 40 % volume Women, 3
Hemoglobin electrophoresis	4	Heparin	Hemoglobi
Hepatitis test (blood)	2	None	Negative

Test	cc. of blood	Acceptable Anticoagulants	Normal Range (Adults)
pH	5	Oiled tube, or heparin	7.35 to 7.45
Phosphatase, acid	5	None	Depends on units, see test.
Phosphatase, alkaline	5	None	Depends on units. *See test.*
Phosphorus	4	None	Adults, 3.0-4.5 mg./100 cc. of serum Children, 4 to 6.5 mg./100 cc. of serum
Plasma electrophoresis for gammopathies	5	None	Comparison to standards
PO_2 (arterial)	Complete tube	Heparin	75 to 95 mm. of mercury
Potassium	6	Oil or none	4 to 5 mEq./L.
Protein (see Albumin)			
Protein-bound iodine (P.B.I.)	8	None	3.0 to 8.0 microgm./100 cc. of serum
Prothrombin time	4.5	Special oxalate solution	11 to 18 seconds = 100%
Red cell fragility	5	Oxalate	Complete hemolysis between 0.30% and 0.36% NaCl (see test)
Salicylates	5	None	None
Sedimentation rate	4	Oxalate, citrate	Men, 0 to 15 mm./hr. Women, 0 to 20 mm./hr. (see test)
Serology	5	None	See test
Sodium	5	Oil or None	138 to 145 mEq./L of serum
Sugar (see Glucose)			
Sulfhemoglobin	5	Oxalate	None
Sulfonamide	5	Oxalate, heparin, E.D.T.A.	None
Thymol turbidity	5	None	Less than 5 units
Thyroxine iodine	6	None	3.0 to 6.4 microgm. per 100 ml. (Murphy & Pattee)
Transaminases SGOT	5	None	10 to 40 units

(Continued)

Test	cc. of blood	Acceptable Anticoagulants	Normal Range (Adults)
SGPT	5	None	5 to 40 units
Urea nitrogen	5	Oxalate, heparin E.D.T.A.	9 to 20 mg./100 cc. of blood
Uric acid	5	Oxalate, heparin E.D.T.A.	2 to 6 mg./100 cc. of serum
Zinc sulfate turbidity	5	None	2 to 12 units

11 Tests Performed on Capillary Blood

(From Finger or Ear Lobe)

Test	Normal Range
Bleeding time	1 to 6 minutes
Guthrie (phenylketonuria)	Negative
Hemoglobin	12 to 18 Gm./100 cc. of blood
Platelet count	200,000 to 500,000/cubic mm. of blood
Red cell count	4 to 6 million/cubic mm. of blood
Reticulocyte count	0.1 to 1.5/100 red blood cells
White cell count	4,000 to 11,000/cubic mm. of blood
White cell differential count	Neutrophiles 54% to 62%
	Eosinophiles 1% to 3%
	Basophiles 0% to 1%
	Lymphocytes 25% to 33%
	Monocytes 0% to 9%

12 Tests Performed on Cerebrospinal Fluid

Test	cc. of Fluid	Normal Range
Chlorides	2	720 to 760 mg. NaCl/100 cc.
Culture	2	Negative
Protein	2	15 to 40 mg./100 cc.
Serology	7	Negative
Sugar	2	50 to 80 mg./100 cc.

Test	Urine Sample	Normal Range
Aceto-acetic acid (see Diacetic Acid)		
Acetone	Random	None
Addis test	12-hr. specimen	Red cells 0 to 450,000 ⎫ White cells 30,000 to 1,000,000 ⎬ † Hyaline casts 0 to 5,000 ⎭
Albumin, qualitative°	Random	None or small amounts
Amino acids	Random or 24-hr.	300 to 650 mgm./24 hr.
Amylase	Timed sample	Under 270 units per hour
Aschheim-Zondek	Morning specimen	Negative
Ascorbic acid tolerance	5 hour sample	Oral - 10% of administered amount Intravenous - 30 to 40% of administered amount
Bacterial count	Clean sample	Under 10,000 per ml.
Bence Jones protein	Random	None
Bile and bilirubin	Random	None
Blood	Random	A few red blood cells (see test)
Calcium (Sulkowitch)	Random	A fine white precipitate
Catecholamines	24-hr. specimen	Less than 140 microgm./24 hrs.
Chlorides, quantitative	24-hr. specimen	See test
Concentration and dilution	Several, at specified intervals (see test)	*Specific gravity* Concentration: 1.026 or higher Dilution: 1.003
Creatinine clearance	24-hr. specimen	100 to 140 ml. per minute
Diacetic (aceto-acetic) acid	Random	None
Fermentation test for sugar	Random	None
Friedman (pregnancy)	Morning specimen	Negative
Frog (pregnancy)	Morning specimen	Negative
Heroin	Special (see morphine)	None
Hogben (pregnancy)	Morning specimen	Negative
Homogentisic acid	Random	None
17-Hydroxycorticosteroids	24-hr. specimen	4 to 12 mgm. in 24 hr.—Differs with other laboratory techniques

°Part of routine urinalysis
†per 12-hr. specimen

Test	Urine Sample	Normal Range
5-Hydroxyindoleacetic acid	24-hr. specimen	Less than 10 mg. in 24 hrs.
Immunologic test for pregnancy	Morning specimen	Negative
17-ketosteroid excretion	24-hr. specimen	Men, 8 to 20 mg./24 hrs. Women, 5 to 15 mg./24 hrs.
Lead	24-hr. specimen	Under 100 mg. in 24 hrs.
Melanin	Random	None
Microscopic°	Random	See test
Morphine	Special (see test)	None
Myoglobin	Random	None
pH°	Random	4.8 to 8.0
Phenolsulfonphthalein (P.S.P.)	Random	Elimination of 63% to 84% in 2 hrs.
Phenylketonuria	Random	None
Porphyrins	24-hr. specimen	Minute amounts
Schilling	See test	See test
Specific gravity°	Random	1.003 to 1.030
Sugar qualitative°	Random	None
Sugar, quantitative	24-hr. specimen	None
Urobilinogen	Differs in different institutions (see test)	Positive reaction at a urine dilution of not more than 1:20
Vanilmandelic acid	24-hr. specimen	Under 7 mg. in 24 hrs.
d-Xylose tolerance (oral)	5-hr. total, minimum 150 cc.	5 to 8 Gm. within 5 hrs. after ingestion

°Part of routine urinalysis

Test	Fecal Specimen	Normal Range
Blood (guaiac or benzidine)	Random, or following meat-free diet, as ordered	May be positive on random specimen
Fat	Random	15% to 25% of weight of dried sample
Parasites	As ordered (see test)	Harmless parasites such as E. coli and flagellates are normal
Undigested food	Random	Small amounts
Urobilin	Random	Large amounts

15   Miscellaneous Tests

Test	Specimen	Normal Range
Gastric analysis, tubeless Basal metabolic rate (B.M.R.)	Patient	—20% to +20%
	Expired air	None
Breath alcohol	Hand (see test)	Light, indistinct hand print
Chloride in sweat	Patient & urine	None
Diatrizoate excretion	Gastric fluid	Depends on stimulus (see test)
Gastric analysis	2-hr. urine specimen (see test)	More than 25 microgm. quinine, or blue color not less than 0.6 mg. azure A standard
Electrocardiogram (E.C.G.)	Patient	Interpretation by cardiologist
Electroencephalogram (E.E.G.)	Patient	Interpretation by neurologist
Microscopic tests for malignant cells	Various body fluids	None
Radioiodine uptake	Patient	20% to 40%
Sputum smears	Sputum	Few eosinophiles or elastic fibers
Thorn	Blood and urine	Eosinophile level fall of at least 50% Uric acid excretion rise of 100%
Thyrotropin	Blood	Not relevant
Tourniquet for capillary fragility	Capillaries of skin of arm	Usually negative

16   Partial List of Drugs and Mixtures Containing Androgens

(Asterisk indicates official or common name)

Adroyd	°Fluoxymesterone	°Methyltestosterone
Anadrol	Formatrix	°Nandrolone
Anavar	Geriatric preparations	Nilevar
Android	(several)	°Norethandrolone
Deca-Durabolin	Gevrestin	Oreton
Depo-Testosterone	Gevrine	°Oxandrolone
Dianabol	Gynetone	°Oxymetholone
°Dromostanolone	Halodrin	Perandren
Dumogran	Halotestin	Ritonic
Dumone	Hovizyme	°Stanozolol
Durabolin	Mediatric	°Testosterone
Eldec	Metandren	Tylosterone
°Ethylestrenol	°Methandriol	Ultandren
Femandren	°Methandrostenolone	Winstrol

17   Partial List of Drugs and Mixtures Containing Azo Dyes

(Asterisk indicates official or common name)

Azo Gantanol	Azo-Sulfurine	Pyridium
Azo Gantrisin	Azotrex	Suladyne
Azolate	Dolonil	Thiosulfil
Azo-Mandelamine	Mallophene	Uremide
Azophene	°Phenazopyridine	Urobiotic

18 Partial List of Drugs and Mixtures Containing Barbiturates

(Asterisk indicates official or common name)

*Allylbarbituris Acid	Eskabarb	*Phenobarbital
Alurate	Eskaphen	Plexonal
Amesec	Ethalyl	*Probarbital
*Amobarbital	Evipal	Prolaire
Amytal	Fiorinal	Quadamine
*Aprobarbital	Halabar	Sandoptal
*Barbital	*Heptabarbital	*Secobarbital
Belladenal	*Hexobarbital	Secodrin
Bellergal	Ilocalm	Seconal
Brevital	Ipral	Seconesin
*Butabarbital	Lotusate	Sibena
*Butallylonal	Luasmin	Solfoserpine
*Butethal	Luminal	Solfoton
Butibel	Medomin	Sombulex
Butiserpine	*Methitural	Spasticol S. A.
Butisol	*Methohexital	Stental
Chardonna	Nembudeine	Surital
Cholan HMB	Nembudonna	Synirin
Codempiral	Nembugesic	*Talbutal
*Cyclobarbital	Nembutal	TCS Tablets
Dainite	Neconal	Tedral
Daprisal	Neocholan	Tepalate
Deltasmyl	Neraval	Tetrasule-S
Delvinal	Nidar	*Thiamylal
Desbutal	*Pentobarbital	*Thiopental
Dexamyl	Pentothal	Tuinal
Donnatal	Percobarb	Veronal
Donnazyme	Pernoston	*Vinbarbital
Empiral	Phanodorn	Zamitol
	Phenaphen	

19 Partial List of Drugs and Mixtures Containing Chloral Hydrate

Aquachloral	Fello-Sed	Noctec
Beta-Chlor	Felsules	Rectules
En-Chlor	Loryl	Somnos
	Noctagetic	

20 Partial List of Drugs and Mixtures Containing Cortisone or its Derivatives

(Asterisk indicates official or common name)

Acne-Cort-Dome	°Desoxycorticosterone	Neo-Hydeltrasol
Alflorone	Dexameth	Neo-Medrol
Alphadrol	°Dexamethasone	Neo-Oxylone
Anusol	Domeform	Neosone
Aquacort	Dronactin	Neo-Synalar
Aristocort	Es-A-Cort	Optef
Aristoderm	F-Cortef	Otobione
Aristogesic	Fernisolone-B	Oxylone
Aristomin	Florinef	Pabalate-HC
Ataraxoid	°Fludrocortisone	Pabirin
Aural acute	°Fluorometholone	Pantho-F
°Betamethasone	Formtone	Paracort
Blephamide	Gammacorten	Paracortol
Caldecort	Haldrone	°Paramethasone
Carbo-Cort	Hexaderm	Percorten
Celestone	Hexadrol	Predne-Dome
Chymar	Hist-A-Cort	Prednefrin
Collosul HC	Hycortole	°Prednisolone
Conjunctilone	Hydeltra	°Prednisone
Cordran	Hydeltrasol	Protef
Cort-Acne	°Hydrocortamate	Rectal Medicone-HC
Cor-Tar-Quin	°Hydrocortisone	Respihaler Decadron
Cortate	Hydrocortone	Respihaler Pro
Cort-Dome	Hytone	Decadron
Cortef	Kenacort	Salcort
Cortifan	Kenalog	Sigmagen
°Cortisol	Ledaform-HC	Solu-Cortef
°Cortisone	Lida-Mantle	Solu-Medrol
Cortogen	Lipo-Adrenal Cortex	Somacort
Cortone	Magnacort	Sterane
Cortril	Medrol	Sterazolidin
Decadron	°Methylprednisolone	Sterne
Decagesic	Meticortetone	Sterolone
Decaspray	Meticorten	Synalar
Decortin	Meti-Derm	Tarcortin
Decosterone	Metimyd	Tenda Cream
Delenar	Metreton	Terra-Cortril
Delta-Cortef	Mycolog	°Triamcinolone
Delta-Dome	Neo-Aristocort	Triamel-HC
Deltasmyl	Neo-Aristoderm	Vio-Fernisone
Deltasone	Neo-Cort-Dome	Vioform-Hydrocorti-

(Continued)

20 Partial List of Drugs and Mixtures Containing Cortisone or its Derivatives

Deltra	Neo-Cortef	sone
Deltrasone	Neo-Decadron	Vio-Hydrosone
Depo-Medrol	Neo-Delta-Cortef	Vytone
Derma Medicone-HC	Neo-Deltef	Ze-Tar-Quin
Deronil		Zetone

21 Partial List of Drugs and Mixtures Containing Estrogens

(Asterisk indicates official or common name)

°Benzestrol	Estinyl	Lutocylol
°Chlorotrianisene	°Estradiol	°Methallenestril
Clusivol	Estradurin	Milprem
Cylogesterin	°Estriol	Ovocylin
Deladumone	°Estrone	PMB
Delestrogen	Femandren	Premarin
Deluteval	Formatrix	Progynon
Depo-Testadiol	Furestrol	Provest
Dicorvin	Gerilets	Quinette
°Diethylstilbesterol	Gevrestin	Sulestrex
°Dinestrol	Gyneton	Tace
Duosterone	Halodrin	Theelin
°Equilenin	°Hexestrol	Ultrogen
°Equilin	Hovizyme	Vallestril

(Asterisk indicates official or common name)
Part A—Therapeutic Agents

Amend's solution	Iodized Petrogen
Arocalcin	Iodo-Ichthyol
Bronchoid, Jr.	Iosalex ointment
Calathesin	Isopropamide Iodide
Calcidrine	Isuprel Compound Elixir
Ceradine	Itrumil
Cher-Iomine	Limodin
Child's Drikof	Lipoiodine
Creodide	°Lugol's solution
Darbid	Milpath
Di-iodo Tyrosine	°Nail polish
°Dough conditioners (some)	Organidin
Endoarsan	Oridine
Entero-Vioform	°Potassium iodide
Entodon	Quadrinal
Feosol powders & tablets	Quin-O-Creme
Floraquin	°Sodium iodide
Iocapral	Tamponets
Iocylate	Thyractin
Iod-Ethamine	°Tincture of iodine
Iodex	Vioform

Part B—Radiographic Contrast Media

Name (Asterisk indicates official or common name)	Period during which all iodine determinations including pro- tein-bound and radioidine up- take will probably be meaningless
°Acetrizoate	2 weeks
Cardiografin	2 weeks
°Chloriodized oil	1 to 5 years
Cholografin	2 to 6 months
Conray	2 to 6 months
Diodrast	2 to 6 months
°Diatrizoate	2 weeks
Dionosil	2 to 6 months
Diprotrizoate	2 weeks
Ethiodol	1 to 5 years
Gastrografin	2 weeks
Hypaque	2 weeks

(Continued)

Part B—Radiographic Contrast Media

°Iodipamide	2 to 6 months
°Iodized oil	1 to 5 years
°Iodoalphionic acid	2 to 6 months
Iodochloral	1 to 5 years
°Iopanoic acid	2 to 6 months
°Iophendylate	1 to 5 years
°Iophenoxic acid	2 to 6 months
°Iodopyracet	2 to 6 months
°Iothalamate	1 to 5 years
°Ipodate	2 to 6 months
Lipiodol	1 to 5 years
Mediopaque	2 weeks
°Meglumine iothalamate	2 to 6 months
Miokon	2 weeks
Neo-ipax	2 weeks
Oragrafin	2 to 6 months
Pantopaque	1 to 5 years
Priodax	2 to 6 months
°Propyliodone	2 to 6 months
Renographin	2 weeks
Salpix	2 to 6 months
Skiodan	2 to 6 months
Telepaque	2 to 6 months
Teridax	2 to 6 months
Thixokon	2 weeks
Urokon	2 weeks
Visciodol	1 to 5 years

23   **Partial List of Drugs and Mixtures Containing Meprobamate**

Appetrol	Equanil	Miltown
Bamadex	Equanitrate	Miltrate
Cyclex	Meprospan	Pathibamate
Deprol	Meprotabs	PMB
Equagesic	Milpath	Prozine
	Milprem	

24 Partial List of Drugs and Mixtures Containing Oxytetracycline

(Asterisk indicates official or common name)

*Oxytetracycline Terra-Cortril	Terramycin	Terrastatin Urobiotic

25 Partial List of Drugs and Mixtures Containing Phenothiazine Derivatives

(Asterisk indicates official or common name)

*Acetylpromazine	*Methotrimeprazine	Sparine
*Acetophenazine	*Methoxypromazine	Stelazine
*Carphenazine	Mornidine	Tacaryl
Chlorphenergan	Neozine	Temaril
*Chlorpromazine	Notensil	Tentone
*Chlorpromethazine	Pacatal	*Thiethylperazine
Combid	Parsidol	*Thioperazine
Compazine	Pernitil	*Thiopropazate
Coplexen	*Perphenazine	*Thioridazine
Dartal	Phenergan	Thoradex
*Diethazine	*Pipamazine	Thorazine
Diparcol	*Prochlorperazine	Tindal
Eskatrol	Proketazine	Torecan
*Ethapropazine	Prolixin	*Trifluoperazine
*Fluphenazine	*Promazine	*Triflupromazine
Largon	*Promethazine	Trilafon
Mellaril	*Propiomazine	*Trimeprazine
*Mepazine	Prozine	Veractil
Mepergan	*Pyrathiazine	Vesprin
*Methdilazine	Pyrrolazote	Vontil

Butiserpazide
Butiserpine
Diupres
Diutensin
Eskaserp
Hydropres
Iphyllin
Metamine
Metatensin
Naquival

Penite
Renese-R
Salutensin
Sandril
Ser-Ap-Es
Serpasil
Serpatilin
Solfoserpine
Unitensen

27 **Partial List of Drugs and Mixtures Containing Salicylates**

(Asterisk indicates official or common name)

°Acetylsalicylic acid
Arlcaps
A.S.A.
Ascodeen
°Aspirin
Bufferin
Codempiral
Coldene
Cordex
Coricidin
Corilin
Daprisal
Darvon Compound
Darvo-Tran
Decagesic
Delenar
Ecotrin
Edrisal
Empiral
Empirin
Emprazil

Equagesic
Excedrin
Fiorinal
Medaprin
°Methyl salicylate
Monacet Compound
Nembu-Gesic
Pabalate
Pabirin
Percobarb
Percodan
Phenaphen
Pyrroxate
Robaxisal
Salcedrox
Salcort
°Salicylate, sodium
Sigmagen
Thephorin-AC
Trancogesic
Zactirin Compound

Index

Index